Advanced Precautions for Today's O.R.

Advanced Precautions for Today's
O.R.

2001 Edition

The Operating Room Professional's Handbook for the Prevention of Sharps Injuries and Bloodborne Exposures

Mark S. Davis, MD, FACOG

SWEINBINDER PUBLICATIONS LLC
Atlanta, Georgia

First Edition 1999
Second Edition 2001

ISBN: 0-9664873-6-2

LCCN: 2001131000

ATTENTION: HOSPITALS, HEALTHCARE NETWORKS, COLLEGES AND UNIVERSITIES, CORPORATIONS, AND PROFESSIONAL ORGANIZATIONS: Quantity discounts are available on bulk purchases of this book for educational and training purposes, fund raising, or gift giving. For information, please contact: Sweinbinder Publications LLC, Post Office Box 11988, Atlanta, GA 30355.

DEDICATION

This book is dedicated to the healthcare workers and patients who acquire infectious diseases through bloodborne exposures each year and to their families, with the hope and belief that such events can and will be prevented by thoughtful planning and constant vigilance.

ACKNOWLEDGMENTS

This book could not have been created without the help, suggestions, and encouragement of numerous people. I would like to express my deep appreciation:

To the surgeons, perioperative nurses, and surgical technologists on the front line who provided creative input.

To the librarians, operating room managers, and administrators at DeKalb Medical Center.

To the national community of professionals in epidemiology, infectious diseases, infection control, and occupational health, whose collective compassion and dedication to keeping both healthcare worker and patient safe helped inspire me to write this book.

And special thanks to Tom Garry for reviewing the manuscript.

And very special thanks to my style editor, Ina Gottlieb, who many years ago taught my children to correctly and creatively use the English language, for reviewing their father's manuscript and creating order out of chaos.

Finally, sincere thanks to my family for their unending patience and support.

HOW TO CONTACT THE AUTHOR

Mark Davis, MD
PO Box 11988
Atlanta, GA 30355
phone: (404) 233-3359
fax: (404) 233-5662
E-mail: msdavismd@aol.com
Web site URL: www.ORprecautions.com

Mark Davis, MD, provides consulting and educational services to hospitals, healthcare institutions, and industry. Readers are encouraged to contact the author with comments and suggestions for future editions.

CONTENTS

SECTION IV.
ADMINISTRATIVE SUPPORT AND INTERACTION

FOREWORD

"Develop a bias for action. Cultivate the habit of focusing simultaneously on patient safety and occupational safety, throughout every procedure. Constantly observe, analyze, learn, communicate, and teach."

—M. Davis; *Advanced Precautions for Today's O.R.*

Surgical health care providers created a standard of excellence in the practice of infection control at the turn of the century when the value of aseptic techniques to prevent wound infections was first demonstrated. In the past decade, awareness of the risk associated with exposure to blood containing HIV ushered in a new era in surgical infection control—one that emphasizes protection of both patients and surgical care providers. Just as patients must be protected from wound contamination and exposure to injured providers' blood, providers must be protected from intraoperative injuries and other exposures to patients' blood.

The operating room is clearly one of the most hazardous environments in the health care delivery system. By definition, surgery is invasive. Instruments that are designed to penetrate the patient's tissue can just as easily injure the provider. Blood is ubiquitous. Speed is essential. Emergencies can occur at any time and interrupt routines. Clinicians are crowded together in a confined space, often with poor lighting and visibility. Cases are often long and fatigue is common. Preventing injuries and exposures under these circumstances is indeed challenging!

The Centers for Disease Control and Prevention (CDC), the Occupational Safety and Health Administration (OSHA), and many professional societies have formulated guidelines and regulations, based on the principles of "universal precautions", to protect health care workers from blood exposures. These important efforts laid the groundwork for practice changes that led to safety improvements in many health care settings, but have not had a major impact in many operating rooms. In fact, the introduction of universal precautions created confusion in the surgical community. Some surgeons interpreted the guidelines to require the use of maximal barrier protection (plastic aprons, face shields, water-resistant foot protection, etc.) for all procedures, regardless of exposure risk. Others felt that universal precautions (sterile gloves, gowns, surgical masks) were already standard practice in surgery and were just not adequate to protect personnel from blood exposures.

In this handbook, Dr. Mark Davis bridges the gap between the principles of universal precautions and the actual practice of safer surgery. His comprehensive exposure prevention strategy is derived from a very credible basis, that of a practicing surgeon, and draws from published epidemiologic investigations, CDC guidelines, his own observations and experience, and most importantly, common sense. A key theme—the entire surgical team shares risk and shares responsibility for safety—makes this an especially useful handbook for all O.R. personnel, regardless of occupational status or duties.

The science of safety in the O.R. has not kept pace with the urgent need for prevention strategies, and many of the specific recommendations found in this handbook have not been evaluated in clinical studies. Nevertheless, the efficacy of some clearly is supported by data: hepatitis B immunization, use of protective gear appropriate to the level of anticipated exposure risk, double-gloving, sharps management, and use of blunt needles, when appropriate. Most others merit at least a trial evaluation, if not immediate implementation.

Achieving safety in the O.R. ultimately depends on the commitment and teamwork of those on the front lines. Advanced Precautions for Today's O.R. provides a framework for creating a strong "bias for action" and leading others, like Dr. Davis, to "observe, analyze, learn, communicate, and teach" the practice of intraoperative safety.

Julie Louise Gerberding, M.D., M.P.H.
Associate Professor of Medicine (Infectious Diseases) and Epidemiology and Biostatistics
University of California, San Francisco and San Francisco General Hospital

PREFACE

From the earliest times, the list of feared surgical complications has included hemorrhage, infection, and thromboembolism. More recently, serious hospital-acquired (nosocomial) bacterial infections, resistant to most antibiotics, have joined the list. Most recently, frequent occupational exposures to increasingly common viral bloodborne pathogens, including HIV and hepatitis C, with resultant infection of healthcare workers and patients, have come to demand our attention. These bloodborne exposures, and the infections they may cause, are extremely costly events which often find their way into the press and—in today's litigious society—the courtroom, thereby multiplying their potential cost many times over.

The surgical environment is unique, making it a challenge to comply with the intent of the Occupational Safety and Health Administration (OSHA) regulations, but it is well worth the effort. The enormous benefits of preventing sharps injuries and bloodborne exposures extend beyond prevention of occupationally acquired infections; cost savings, liability prevention and stress reduction also define the safe surgical workplace.

OSHA's Compliance Directive (CPL 2-2.44D), effective OSHA-wide November 5, 1999, directs its field inspectors to cite employers (which could include hospitals, physicians and/or their professional corporations) for failure to eliminate or minimize occupational exposure to blood. Stated recommendations for safe practice include implementing work practices such as "no-hands passing" of sharps, and effective engineering controls such as blunt suture needles, where applicable, in order to prevent percutaneous injuries before, during, or after use through safer design features. For more on the Compliance Directive and the Federal Needlestick Safety and Prevention Act (S 3067) adopted by the U.S. Congress in October, 2000, see Appendix C.

Of the bloodborne pathogens most likely to be encountered during surgery—hepatitis B, hepatitis C, and HIV—the only one for which a vaccine is available is hepatitis B, ironically the least potentially lethal of the three. Universal Precautions and Standard Precautions have not, and cannot, come close to eliminating the large numbers of sharps injuries and bloodborne exposures commonly associated with surgical procedures. Focusing on individual preventive measures as well as teamwork, this book was written to help operating room professionals create a safer surgical environment through avoidance of exposures to blood and bloodborne pathogens. The required changes in technique and technology are relatively minor, but the goal of exposure prevention must be kept in clear focus during every invasive procedure. Every institution would be well served by adopting an integrated strategy to take control of these costly adverse events.

In the preface to the nineteenth edition of *Williams Obstetrics*, the reader is wisely counseled, "Obstetrics is art and science combined, and its practitioners must be concerned with the lives of at least two intricately woven patients—the mother and her fetus . . . it is apparent that the responsibility of the obstetrician is enormous." Similarly, the responsibility of today's operating room professionals extends beyond concern for the life of the patient to the lives of fellow care givers who are intricately woven together as a surgical team.

The approach outlined in this book is simple. Because I have tried to be observant while operating, I have identified dangerous and safe ways to function in the surgical environment. Information was additionally gathered from a review of the current literature and discussions with respected surgical colleagues and other frontline healthcare workers. There may be additional appropriate ways to function safely; this book describes some approaches that have been extremely helpful.

Some of the suggestions in this book will be familiar, and you may already be using some of them. The key to success is applying these principles in an integrated and consistent manner. It requires daily attention to detail, persistence and determination. You will face the obstacles of inertia, denial, and cost containment at your institution, but these can be overcome by sufficient teamwork and education.

There is arguably nothing more frightening for a healthcare worker than to learn he or she has been exposed to HIV and then having to wait months to find out if he or she has become infected. Understanding we cannot eliminate risk entirely, those of us at DeKalb Medical Center who use the techniques and protocols described in this book have nevertheless been able to reduce our occupational risk and the accompanying anxiety. Truly, our lives have changed.

A set of *Advanced Precautions*—selection and deployment of the most effective (and cost-effective) currently available personal protective equipment, safety devices, and safety protocols—are described in this book. This information is directly applicable to the clinical setting. Like the deadly pathogens that inspired them, whatever precautions we select will need to evolve over time to remain successful. They must be monitored, maintained, and upgraded by a process of continuous quality improvement.

As individuals and surgical team members, we must try to simultaneously create a safer environment for both the surgical patient and the surgical team. We are involved in a continual learning process; as knowledge deepens and technology evolves, this handbook will be updated appropriately. Readers are encouraged to share with the author their successes, as well as their persistent problems.

A complaint commonly heard—and one of the frustrating challenges to any institution—stems from individuals who are not sufficiently committed to changing the system. As more and more people learn to use safer techniques and technology, the position of the minority who do not becomes more difficult to justify and defend.

Finally, OSHA regulations and employer responsibilities aside, remember it is *your* workplace and yours to change. By the choices you make, you take considerable control of your own destiny. Protect yourself first; then plan to work safely as a team. Visualize a safer workplace and share that vision with your co-workers. Be a vocal advocate for safety and lead by example.

Your attention will be diverted at times by other problems but, above all, be persistent. If you consistently follow an integrated system for exposure prevention such as the one found in this book, it will work for you and your co-workers.

I wish you much success.

MSD

Why This Book Was Written

The Awakening

What prompted a busy obstetrician/gynecologic surgeon after 25 years of practice to write a book on occupational safety for operating room professionals? In the late 1980s, I was severely cut with a scalpel while performing a hysterectomy. This was when we were just becoming aware of the significance of the silently spreading HIV/AIDS epidemic. Interviewing the patient in the recovery room, I was shocked and surprised to learn of some risk factors in her husband's lifestyle. Those factors placed both of us at risk and we had to be tested for HIV.

Although the tests were negative, I replayed the events of the injury in my mind and realized the accident could have been prevented had there been a plan in place to manage sharps more safely. Personal safety had not been addressed during my training and all I had learned were the habits, good and bad, of my mentors. In the complex, confined, and volatile environment of the operating room where things often happen unexpectedly, simply being careful had not prevented the injury. I had learned a powerful and valuable lesson. The subconscious denial of risk had been erased, and this freed me to focus on seeking solutions to the problem.

By the early 1990s, general perception of the magnitude of the HIV epidemic had increased, and by the mid-1990s, another potentially lethal bloodborne pathogen, hepatitis C, was capturing the attention of epidemiologists and surgeons. It was becoming increasingly clear the causes for the many occupational exposures being reported needed to be defined and practices developed to reduce these risks.

Life-Changing Experiences

I attended and participated in several national and international conferences dealing with the prevention of sharps injuries and bloodborne exposures, meeting with others concerned with the problem. I met a nurse and a physician who had become occupationally infected with HIV and heard their heartbreaking stories of preventable needlestick injuries, which had resulted in seroconversion. I sensed their rage and frustration. At that time, a physician who was a good friend and colleague of mine died of chronic hepatitis C, despite a successful liver transplant.

The Search for Answers

I needed to find ways in which to make the operating room a safer workplace. Knowing that most sharps injuries are caused by suture needles and having had my skin and gloves punctured by suture needles many times, I began studying and testing a new generation of blunt-tipped suture needles that had just become commercially available. They appeared to be effective in preventing needlesticks and glove tears without causing harm to patients. After evaluating every available brand and size of blunt-tipped suture needles for gynecological surgery and operative obstetrics and determining where and how to use them most effectively, I began to use them routinely. By almost totally avoiding the most commonly used sharp instrument in surgery, the traditional sharp suture needle, I found I was able to eliminate much of the hazard associated with suturing. What made it even better was not only was I protected, but so was every member of the surgical team.

By constantly focusing on safety in the operating room, regularly reviewing available literature, evaluating new safety-engineered devices, speaking and consulting at hospitals, and exchanging views and ideas with surgeons from around the world, I was able to collect and refine a number of useful techniques. I soon realized there were many underutilized techniques, devices, and strategies that could be implemented to decrease the risk of exposure. That knowledge, synthesized into an integrated system for exposure prevention, became the basis for this book.

The information herein needs to be shared.

Who Should Read This Book?

Those at Occupational Risk

In addition to inpatient and outpatient operating rooms and ambulatory surgery centers, operative procedures are commonly performed in patient rooms, emergency departments, intensive care and coronary care units, interventional radiology and physician offices. This handbook was written to help create and maintain a safer working environment for every member of the surgical team and in a larger sense, for everyone who may perform in the operative environment, including:

- Surgeons
- Residents
- Obstetricians
- Midwives
- Anesthesia personnel
- Perioperative nurses
- Surgical assistants
- Surgical technologists
- Labor and delivery nurses
- Obstetrical technologists
- Medical students
- Nursing students
- Technology students
- CRNA students
- Emergency Department personnel
- Radiology personnel
- Intensive Care personnel
- Pathologists

Others Who Can Help

A concurrent objective of this book is to facilitate and assure compliance with OSHA's requirements in two particularly hazardous work sites: the operating room and the delivery room, as well as the other work sites listed above. Hospital administrators and managers at various levels will benefit from reading this book, including:

- Surgical services directors
- Operating room managers
- Obstetrical service managers
- Risk managers
- Materials managers
- Infection control team
- Occupational health team
- CQI and quality assurance teams
- Workers compensation and insurance providers

All of these people in the hospital organization have critical roles to play in facilitating exposure prevention. Risk managers and materials managers, in particular, need to have a firm understanding of the scope and complexity of hazards found in the surgical setting and should read the chapters in the first section of this book as well as other appropriate chapters to visualize the big picture. Doing so will facilitate well-informed purchasing decisions that optimally serve both the institution and healthcare workers at risk.

How to Use This Book
Understanding Risks and Identifying Problems

Section I (chapters 1 through 3) provides an overview of the problem and a broad perspective, including a review of the incidence of occupational transmission of HIV and the common hepatic viruses. Adverse consequences and costs resulting from bloodborne exposures are surveyed and causes of sharps injuries and bloodborne exposures are identified.

Identifying Solutions and Facilitating Change

Sections II and III (chapters 4 through 14) show an integrated system for exposure prevention—a head-to-toe how-to-choose and how-to-use approach—with comprehensive descriptions of safety protocols, safe surgical techniques, personal protective equipment, and choices of safer technology. Section IV (chapters 15 through 18) suggests ways in which managerial staff and administration may successfully interact with those at risk to facilitate exposure prevention. Chapter 17 also provides guidelines for conducting effective product evaluations.

Three appendices are included. Appendix A provides a detailed model Safety Checklist intended for daily use that may be copied and posted on or near the door of every operating room and delivery room. The checklists serve as safety reminders and as a means of raising awareness of risk among personnel. Checklists should be tailored to procedures and personnel and regularly reviewed and updated as new technology and techniques evolve.

Appendix B provides the most current recommendations (at the time of publication) for managing occupational exposures. O.R. professionals need to know how to respond promptly in the event of an occupational exposure. They should understand in advance the process of post-exposure management. Such an understanding in itself is a safety motivating factor. Infection control professionals and others caring for exposed workers will be on a learning curve for some time to come as data are collected on the efficacy and toxicity of drugs used for HIV post-exposure prophylaxis. Guidelines will change frequently. Use the section, Additional Educational Resources, to access updated protocols via web sites and other listings.

Appendix C provides a summary of OSHA regulations relevant to the operating room, including the Compliance Directive of November, 1999. Operating room professionals should know what the law requires and what the OSHA guidelines are. The guidelines make it clear those at risk must make more specific safer choices of equipment and protocols to realize an effective exposure prevention plan.

Space is provided at the end of each chapter for notation of real or potential hazards you may identify specific to your work site and your planned corrective measures. Think of it not as a blank page for notes, but a powerful tool for implementing change. It is suggested this book be kept in the hospital locker and/or at the nursing station, readily accessible for reference and notation.

An index, a glossary, and additional educational resources are also provided. References and suggested readings appear at the end of chapters, where appropriate.

Author's Plea to Fellow Surgeons

As the "captain of the ship," the daily repetitive and habitual choices we make when we ask for scalpels, sutures, and other sharp devices have the potential of positively or negatively impacting the lives of many— the patient, ourselves, those standing across from or next to us at the operating table, others working in the room, and the families of all.

Accordingly, although I may feel as competent using a sharp suture needle versus a blunt one for most suturing tasks, I also know despite the fact everyone tries to be careful, needlesticks occur in unacceptable numbers. Once an accident happens, uncontrollable negative forces are set in motion. There is immediate major stress and anxiety. Toxic drugs may have to be taken. Seroconversion, *the unthinkable*, looms as a possibility. One of the things I do, therefore, is to routinely choose the blunt suture needle in preference to the sharp whenever possible to protect myself and the other people involved.

Because of choices I have made, my life has changed: I enjoy operating more and I sleep better at night. Everyone in the operating room is glad to see me and people want to scrub on my cases. Responsible for the choices of safer devices and protocols, surgeons have become custodians of the well being of an extended group of people beyond the patient. Like spoken words that cannot be retrieved, the seemingly trivial decisions we make many times a day may return to haunt . . . or to bless us.

Think carefully before you choose.*

*Editor's note: Since the publication of the first edition of this handbook in March, 1999, OSHA has clarified its position on the need to implement some of the safety devices and practices described herein. This is reinforced by the Federal Needlestick Safety and Prevention Act (S 3067) adopted by the U.S. Congress in October, 2000. See OSHA Compliance Directive, Appendix C.

SECTION I

Overview
and
Perspective

CHAPTER 1

Bloodborne Pathogens and Occupational Risk

The Problem

Any successful program for managing the occupational risk of exposure to bloodborne pathogens must be predicated upon understanding the scope of the problem. The most common bloodborne pathogens of concern to operating room professionals are hepatitis B, hepatitis C, and HIV. According to OSHA's Final Rule, published in 1991, more than 4 million healthcare workers in the United States are considered at risk of occupational infection.

The hepatitis B vaccination has dramatically reduced the threat to healthcare workers from that disease, but it has not eliminated it. Not everyone at risk has been vaccinated, and some individuals do not produce an adequate antibody response following vaccination.

Hepatitis C, often a silent and chronic disabling disease, is highly infectious via percutaneous exposure, and there is no vaccine or post-exposure prophylaxis. While HIV and AIDS initially captured most of the attention regarding occupational exposures, hepatitis C is arguably of more concern to operating room professionals and patients in the new millennium.

HIV will remain an occupational risk to O.R. professionals with global spread of the epidemic and evolution of strains of virus resistant to antiretroviral medications. Despite the routine use of gloves and protective apparel (Universal Precautions), large numbers of exposures continue to be reported. As of the end of 1997, an estimated 30 million persons worldwide were infected with HIV; of these, approximately 40% were women and 1 million were children under the age of 15. Only an estimated 10% of infected individuals are aware of their condition.

The Solution

The approach to reducing the risk of exposure to any one of these bloodborne infectious agents must address all three, as well as other evolving infectious agents. Hospital occupational health departments document a wide variety of injury and exposure scenarios, but injury and exposure patterns may be site-specific and recurrent with individuals. The problem could be frequent glove failure, needlestick injury, mucous membrane exposure, or any combination. In this era of evolving bloodborne pathogens, the fundamental goal for operating room professionals is to prevent contact with the blood of all patients. To effectively reduce occupational risk, an advanced integrated strategy that takes full advantage of safety engineered devices, safety protocols, and safe work practices must be consistently applied.

Patients and Care Givers Share the Risk

The opportunities for bloodborne transmission of infectious agents are bidirectional. A *surgical exposure* is here defined as contact between blood of an injured surgeon or other member of the surgical team—caused by scalpels, needles, or other sharp devices—and the internal tissues of a surgical patient. The CDC refers to this as a *recontact*. Recent reports from the US, the UK, and Spain have documented surgeons infected with hepatitis B and hepatitis C, acquired from patients by previous occupational bloodborne exposures, may transmit these infections to surgical patients.

The French National Public Health Network has reported a case of transmission of HIV from an orthopedic surgeon to a patient. Further investigation revealed that the surgeon sustained frequent sharps injuries and was not aware of his own advanced HIV infection. The case of the Florida dentist who transmitted HIV to several of his patients is widely known, but numerous retrospective studies have thus far failed to reveal any other instances of HIV transmission from dentists, surgeons, and other healthcare workers to patients. Despite these isolated reports, transmission of HIV to patients from surgeons is, therefore, considered extremely unlikely if appropriate precautions are taken in exposure-prone invasive settings.

Restriction of Surgical Privileges

In the United Kingdom, healthcare workers infected with bloodborne pathogens are restricted from participating in invasive procedures. In the United States, hospital safety and infection control committees may, at their discretion, restrict infected healthcare personnel from participating in invasive procedures. By adopting appropriate and effective precautions, operating room professionals can simultaneously protect themselves and their patients.

Infectious Blood and Body Fluids

Universal Precautions (see also Standard Precautions, below) originally defined the infectious materials encountered in operative settings as follows.

Highest risk:
- Blood
- Fluids containing visible blood
- Wound drainage or exudates

Others:
- Semen
- Vaginal secretions
- Tissues
- Cerebrospinal fluid
- Sputum
- Synovial fluid
- Pleural fluid
- Peritoneal fluid
- Amniotic fluid
- Feces

Universal Precautions did not apply to the following materials unless blood is visibly present:
- Tears
- Nasal secretions
- Saliva
- Sweat
- Urine
- Vomit

It is possible, however, for blood to be present in minute quantities without being visible. In such cases, if the blood has a high viral content (viral load), exposed workers may still be at significant risk of infection.

Standard Precautions

Standard Precautions were defined and issued by the Centers for Disease Control and Prevention (CDC) and the Hospital Infection Control Practices Advisory Committee (HICPAC) in 1996. They combine Universal Precautions and Body Substance Isolation. The latter was designed to reduce the risk of transmission of pathogens from moist body substances. Standard Precautions apply to blood, *all* body fluids, secretions, and excretions (*except sweat*), regardless of whether they contain visible blood. Intended to protect nonintact skin and mucous membranes, Standard Precautions are designed to reduce the risk of transmission of microorganisms from both recognized and unrecognized sources of infection in hospitals. It is logical, prudent, and hygienic to wear gloves when working with any and all body fluids.

Hepatitis B Virus (HBV)

Hepatitis B virus is transmissible by needlestick in up to 30% of exposures to infectious sources; 5 to 10% of HBV infections become chronic. Fatal acute fulminant hepatitis occurs in less than 1% of cases, but months of disability may result from acute hepatitis B infection, and the potential for spread to family members is high. Fortunately, HBV is preventable in most cases by vaccination.

Hepatitis B Vaccination

All operating room professionals are at risk of contact with blood and should be vaccinated against hepatitis B. Workers who are eligible for the vaccine and have not received it place themselves and their families at unnecessary risk. The vaccines are safe and well tolerated. There is no risk of HIV infection from modern genetically engineered vaccines. Mild soreness at the injection site for one to two days may occur in up to 20% of persons. Occasionally, fatigue, headache, or fever may occur, but there have been no severe acute or chronic adverse effects reported due to vaccination. According to the CDC, the duration of protection following vaccination is at least 14 years and studies continue. Vaccines are provided by employers at no cost to healthcare workers at risk of exposure to blood, as mandated by OSHA regulations.

Three doses of 1 milliliter of vaccine are given intramuscularly at 0 month, 1 month, and 6 months, preferably in the deltoid muscle. Vaccine recipients over the age of 30, those with impaired immune response, and those who received the vaccine in the buttock rather than the deltoid muscle may not sufficiently respond with adequate antibody formation. The series of three doses of vaccine, when given as above, is effective in more than 95% of otherwise healthy young adults who respond to the vaccination. Post-vaccination testing to demonstrate sufficient antibody formation appears to be a cost-effective precaution, as this may eliminate the need for booster injections following an exposure years later when antibodies may have fallen to undetectable levels. Up to three additional doses should be administered to persons who don't respond to the initial series; about 50% will respond.

A small percentage of people will not respond sufficiently to the vaccine to prevent infection following exposure (nonresponders), and post-exposure prophylaxis with HBIG (hepatitis B immune globulin) is required in such cases. (For a more detailed discussion of vaccination, see Appendix B.)

Hepatitis C Virus (HCV)

First identified in 1989, hepatitis C has emerged as a highly significant occupational health risk to operating room professionals. Healthcare workers are at an estimated 20-40 fold greater risk occupationally from HCV than HIV. Of the estimated 400,000 health care worker sharps injury exposures in the acute care setting annually in the US, 20,000 to 30,000 are to HCV. Of those exposed health care workers, 500 to 700 will acquire the disease. Hepatitis C is the most common chronic bloodborne infection in the US. Healthcare workers face greater exposure and disease risks as the prevalence of HCV in the patient base increases. HCV is the cause of half of chronic liver disease deaths each year; chronic liver disease being the 10th leading cause of death among adults in the US. (Source: Frontline Healthcare Workers Safety Conference, Aug. 6-8, 2000 Washington, DC.)

As of 1997, there were approximately 4.5 million reported hepatitis C infections in the United States, representing 1.8% of the general population, with 2,200 infections reported in healthcare workers. Seropositivity rates in hospital personnel range from 1.4 to 5.5%. Studies of the prevalence of HCV in hospital patients vary, but up to 18% of emergency room patients may harbor the virus. Transmission of hepatitis C infection from patients to healthcare workers has been documented as a result of accidental needlesticks or cuts with sharp instruments, as well as from a blood splash to the conjunctiva. The risk of occupational infection with HCV following percutaneous injury has been reported to be from 3% to as high as 10%, depending on the accuracy of the methods used for testing and the viral load in the source patient. The latest CDC estimate is 2% to 3%.

The human host produces an ineffective immune response to HCV. The rate of chronic infection (85%) is extremely high compared to hepatitis B. Because HCV mutates rapidly, multiple exposures to subtypes of HCV may yield multiple opportunities for infection and reinfection. About 20% of persons chronically infected with HCV will develop end-stage cirrhosis, liver failure, or liver cancer. HCV is the leading cause for liver transplantation in the U.S. In no case does liver transplantation rid the host of virus, and newly transplanted livers may become infected and decompensate more rapidly than with the original infection. When this occurs, patients are not considered candidates for repeat liver transplantation. There are an estimated 8,000 to 10,000 deaths from HCV each year, and mortality is expected to triple in the next 10 to 20 years without effective intervention.

Although 250 healthcare workers (HCWs) die annually from hepatitis B (HBV), the long-term lethal potential of hepatitis C in HCWs is projected to be much greater because of the high rate of chronic infection. HCV is found with increased frequency in patients with HIV, and simultaneous transmission of both pathogens has been reported following an exposure. In that instance, the infected HCW died rapidly from liver disease.

There is no vaccine for HCV, nor is it likely one will be produced anytime soon because of the tendency of the virus to mutate frequently. Unlike with HIV, there is no post-exposure prophylaxis for HCV. Medical treatment of HCV (with interferon) is expensive, has many adverse effects, is ineffective in the majority of patients, and has a high relapse rate when the drug is discontinued. Treatment with other drugs and drug combinations is currently being evaluated in clinical trials. In June, 1998 the Federal Drug Administration (FDA) approved the combination therapy interferon with ribavirin for patients 18 years or older with compensated liver disease due to hepatitis C who have relapsed after initial treatment with interferon. Combination therapy may be extended to individuals with early infection to prevent chronic hepatitis. In spite of any benefits of early treatment, the lifetime cost of care for a hepatitis C patient is projected to be from $200,000 to $400,000, with an additional cost of $400,000 for a liver transplant.

Although the mode of transmission of HCV is mainly bloodborne, in more than 40% of HCV-infected patients there is no obvious route of transmission found. In up to 13% of cases, HCV may be acquired through household or family contact, placing families of infected healthcare workers at risk. Given these sobering statistics, the only currently available strategy to reduce the occupational hazard of HCV is the universal avoidance of exposure to blood.

Human Immunodeficiency Virus (HIV)

The epidemic spread of HIV has heightened awareness of this virus as an occupational risk factor for healthcare workers. The first case of occupational transmission of HIV infection was reported in 1984. Through September 1993, 120 healthcare workers had been reported to the CDC as having occupationally acquired AIDS/HIV infection. Of these, 39 were considered by the CDC as documented, and 81 were considered possibly occupationally acquired. Through December 1996, the number of documented cases reported to the CDC had risen from 39 to 52 and the number of possibly occupationally acquired cases had risen from 81 to 111. By December, 1999, the number of documented cases in the US had reached 56 and the number of possible cases 136. More than 80% of cases of occupationally acquired HIV infections in healthcare workers were the result of sharps injuries.

In one year there were at least 500,000 reported injuries due to contaminated needlesticks and other sharp objects. Of these, an estimated 16,000 may have been HIV-contaminated. Most involved hollow-bore needles. According to various studies, HIV seroprevalence in hospital and surgical patients may vary from 0.5 to 23% or more in urban centers. A prospective study showed a majority of sharps injuries and mucocutaneous exposures to blood occurring in the operative setting were not reported, and most involved suture needles. CDC officials have voiced the following concern: incomplete data on exposures in surgery due to incomplete reporting limits their ability to define the risk of seroconversion in operative settings.

The risk of seroconversion to HIV following hollow needlesticks is 0.3% on average, but risk is significantly increased in the following cases: where the source patient has very advanced AIDS, where the needle was visibly contaminated with blood, and where the needle had been used in an artery or vein before the exposure occurred. Post-exposure prophylaxis with zidovudine (ZDV) has been shown to significantly decrease the risk of seroconversion but may be less effective in the presence of increased risk factors. Two, or possibly three, antiretroviral drugs may be offered in exposures considered high risk. (See Appendix B for post-exposure prophylaxis guidelines and information on how to obtain updates.)

The average risk of seroconversion to HIV following suture needlesticks is thought to be significantly lower than with hollow-bore needles, but this risk is more difficult to define because of incomplete reporting of suture needle injuries. As the titer of HIV in blood (viral load) increases, the risk of seroconversion increases. The incidence of sharps injuries during surgical procedures has been reported to be as high as 15% when dedicated observers are used to monitor procedures, and the majority of reported sharps injuries in operative settings are from suture needlesticks.

The CDC estimates the risk of seroconversion to HIV after mucous membrane or nonintact skin exposure is 0.1%, and the risk of seroconversion after intact skin exposure is less than 0.1%. As with needlesticks, these are average risk calculations. The incidence of mucocutaneous exposure to blood during a surgical procedure has been observed to be as high as 40 to 50%.

If one considers the operating room professional's 30-year-career risk of occupationally acquiring HIV by factoring in the number of sharps injuries per year (most of which go unreported), the projected rise in the percentage of surgical patients harboring HIV in the future and the potential for multidrug-resistant strains of HIV, one's perception of risk increases. As with hepatitis C, universal prevention of exposure to blood is the paramount strategy for reducing the risk of occupational transmission of HIV.

HIV Post-Exposure Prophylaxis

The most current recommendations published by the CDC can be found in Appendix B. Guidelines for treatment of occupationally exposed healthcare workers with antiretroviral medications will continue to evolve as experience is gained regarding the efficacy and toxicity of various drugs and drug combinations. Epidemiologists are concerned that, unless and until a vaccine against HIV is produced, we are caught in a race between finding new and better antiretroviral prophylaxis drugs and the development of drug-resistant strains of HIV.

Hepatitis D (HDV)

Hepatitis D is a defective virus that is unable to replicate in the human host without binding to hepatitis B virus. Infections with HDV are generally more severe than with HBV alone, and chronic HBV carriers with HDV superinfection have a 70% incidence of developing chronic liver disease with cirrhosis. Vaccination against hepatitis B protects against HDV.

Other Bloodborne Infectious Diseases

Tuberculosis and other serious infectious diseases have been transmitted to healthcare workers through percutaneous exposure. Bloodborne M. tuberculosis is found with increased frequency in patients with HIV, and the emergence of drug-resistant strains of tuberculosis has become an additional cause for concern. Rarely seen agents such as the Ebola virus and malaria could be spread by occupational exposure to blood, as could a long list of other serious but uncommon diseases. It is neither the purpose nor the scope of this book to consider all of these in detail, but an important point can be made: If O.R. professionals use an integrated strategy to deal with the common bloodborne pathogens HIV, HCV, and HBV, little or no adjustments will be necessary when faced with operating on patients with exotic diseases.

Estimated Annual Health Care Worker Infections

The CDC estimates that 400 new occupational HBV infections occurred in 1995 among U.S. health care workers, down from 17,000 in 1983. (Arch Intern Med 1997;157:2601-2603)

Assuming that between 1% and 2% of patients are HIV-positive (and therefore that 1% to 2% of needlesticks are HIV-contaminated) between 18 to 35 new occupational HIV infections would occur from percutaneous injuries each year. Infections resulting from blood exposures to non-intact skin or mucuous membranes would add between 2 to 4 cases (based on a transmission rate of .09% for a mucous membrane exposure).

Assuming that between 2% and 10% of patients are HCV-positive (Dr. Richard Garvin, Hepatitis Branch, CDC), between 59 to 1,180 new occupational HCV infections would occur each year. Infections resulting from blood exposures to non-intact skin or mucous membranes would add between 16 to 393 cases (assuming that the transmission rate was between 0.4% and 2% per exposure, with lower limit from Dr. Giuseppe Ippolito, Italy, 1999). Source: EPINet. (Data presented at the 2000 Frontline Healthcare Workers Safety Conference project an estimated 500 to 700 occupational HCV infections annually.)

Unreported Injuries and Exposures

Although the focus of this book is prevention, exposures cannot be totally eliminated. If despite our best efforts an exposure occurs, it should be reported. While reporting and post-exposure follow-up does generate anxiety, nonreporting generates both anxiety and denial and could lead to disastrous consequences. In the case of significant exposure to HIV, initiation of post-exposure prophylaxis should begin as soon as possible, preferably within one to two hours, according to the U.S. Public Health Service (see Appendix B). Timely and accurate data collection following an exposure helps to ensure the exposed healthcare worker receives prompt and appropriate treatment and a clearly outlined course of follow-up.

Workers are more likely to report if a well-established and known plan is in place. Currently, computerized self-reporting systems are being developed to facilitate immediate and direct reporting by the exposed worker, preserve confidentiality, and facilitate appropriate counseling and follow-up.

References/Suggested Readings

Alter MJ. Epidemiology of hepatitis C in the west. *Semin Liver Dis* 1995;15:5–14.

Andreone P, Gramenzi A, Cursaro C, et al. Familial cluster of hepatitis C virus type 1. *J Infect Dis* 1994;170:1042–1043.

Cardo DM, Culver DH, Ciesielski CA, Srivastava PU, Marcus R, Abiteboul D, Heptonstall J, Ippolito G, Lot F, McKibben PS, Bell DM, and the Centers for Disease Control and Prevention Needlestick Surveillance Group. A case-control study of HIV seroconversion in health care workers after percutaneous exposure. *NEJM* 1997;337:1485-1490.

Centers for Disease Control and Prevention. Public Health Service Guidelines for the Management of Health-Care Worker Exposure to HIV and Recommendations for Post-exposure Prophylaxis. MMWR 1998;47(No. RR-7):[Inclusive page numbers].

Centers for Disease Control and Prevention: *HIV/AIDS Surveillance Report* 1993;5(3):13.

Esteban JI, Gomez J, Marlett M, et al. Transmission of hepatitis C virus by a cardiac surgeon. *NEJM 1996*;334:555–560.

Grady, GF, Lee VA, Prince AM, et al. Hepatitis B immune globulin for accidental exposures among medical personnel: Final report of a multicenter controlled trial. *J Infect Dis* 1978;138:625.

Jagger J, Pearson D. Universal precautions: still missing the point on needlesticks. *Infect Control Hosp Epidemiol* 1991;12:211–213.

Kao JH, Chen PJ, Lai MY, Chen DS. Superinfection of heterologous hepatitis C virus in patient with chronic type C hepatitis. *Gastroenterology* 1993;105:583–587.

Kelen GD, Green GB, Purcell RH, et al. Hepatitis B and Hepatitis C in emergency room patients. *NEJM* 1992;326:1399–1404.

Lanphear BO, Linneman CC, Cannon CG. Hepatitis C virus infection in healthcare workers: risk of exposure and infection. *Infect Control Hosp Epidemiol* 1994;15:745–750.

Lynch P, White MC. Perioperative blood contact and exposures: a comparison of incident reports and focused studies. *Am J Infect Control* 1993;212:357–363.

MMWR 1995 Dec 22;44(50):929-933. Case-control study of HIV seroconversion in health-care workers after percutaneous exposure to HIV-infected blood—France, United Kingdom, and United States January 1988-August 1994.

MMWR 1996 June 9;45:468–472 Center for Disease Control and Prevention. Update: provisional recommendations for chemoprophylaxis after occupational exposure to HIV.

MMWR 1991;40:1 Centers for Disease Control: Hepatitis B virus: A comprehensive strategy for eliminating transmission in the United States through universal childhood vaccination: Recommendations of the Immunization Practices Advisory Committee (ACIP).

National Institutes of Health Consensus Development Conference Panel Statement: Management of hepatitis C. *Hepatology* 26 (suppl. 1):25-105, 1997.

Quebbeman EJ, Telford GL, Hubbard S, et al. Risk of blood contamination and injury to operating room personnel. *Ann Surg* 1991;214:614–620.

Ridzon R, Gallagher K, Ciesielski C, et al. Simultaneous transmission of HIV and HCV from a needlestick injury. *NEJM* 1997;336:919–922.

Sartori M, La Terra G, Aghetta M, et al. Transmission of hepatitis C via blood splash into conjunctiva. *Scand J Infect Dis* 1993;25:270–271.

The Incident Investigation Teams et al. Transmission of hepatitis B to patients from four infected surgeons without hepatitis B e antigen. *NEJM* 1997;336:178–184.

Tokars JI, Chamberland ME, Schable CA, et al. A survey of occupational blood contact and HIV infection among orthopedic surgeons. *JAMA* 1992;268:489.

Notes

CHAPTER 2

Direct and Indirect Costs of Injuries and Exposures

Injuries and exposures are a threat not only to the health and safety of healthcare workers but are likely to have a far-ranging impact on healthcare organizations. The direct cost of initial follow-up of an exposure (laboratory, vaccines, medications, supplies, and staff time) may be as much as $3,500. A recent study compared costs in two large hospitals, one a community hospital in a high-HIV prevalence region and the other a teaching hospital in a low-HIV prevalence region. The costs in both hospitals were similar.

Addressing the direct cost of exposures on a national scale, there are 30 million surgical procedures performed annually in the US. It has been shown 7 to 15% of surgeries are associated with needlesticks or other sharps injuries when dedicated observers are stationed in the operating room to record them rather than relying on workers to report their injuries. Using a rounded average of 10%, this yields 2.6 million injuries annually, both reported and unreported. If one multiplies only the estimated 800,000 reported injuries involving contaminated sharps times $1500 (a conservative figure), one finds $1,200,000,000 may be spent annually by the healthcare system for initial follow-up of reported bloodborne exposures. Data collected by EPINet indicate that hospitals experience on average 30 exposures per 100 hospital beds annually. Using these figures, a 300 bed hospital might spend $135,000 ($1500x90) annually. In the year 2000 many hospitals were able to reduce the incidence of sharps injury through the introduction of needleless systems and shielded or retractable needles for injection and

21

vascular access in non-surgical worksites. *This has left the OR as the chief source of injury in 2001.*

These figures, however, are only the tip of the iceberg as they do not reflect the potential costs incurred by the following indirect costs:

- Time lost from work because of illness or disability
- Psychiatric counseling for exposed healthcare workers
- Drugs used for HIV prophylaxis or to treat acquired infections
- Workers compensation payments
- Replacement and training of personnel
- Liability claims lost, settled, or defended
- OSHA fines

It is not difficult to envision the lifetime cost of a single exposure resulting in seroconversion to HIV or hepatitis C easily reaching seven figures. Payments from health insurance and disability insurance may be limited in many cases, leaving the infected individual and his or her family with the additional burden of residual healthcare costs.

Additionally, workers compensation laws, as currently written, may not compensate workers occupationally infected with HIV and other bloodborne pathogens. If benefits do apply at all, they may be woefully insufficient to compensate for the damage done. Bloodborne exposures can also create stress and burnout, prompting much-needed health care professionals to drop out and making it difficult to recruit replacements. It is easy to see that the overall impact of bloodborne exposures on healthcare institutions can be devastating.

The Human Cost

In addition to the dollar cost incurred by bloodborne exposures, one must consider the human cost. Anyone who has gone through post-exposure management of having to wait six months to a year for the return of HIV test results understands this. The emotional toll to the injured worker and the family from stress and restrictions on sex, attempting pregnancy, or breast feeding can be devastating. In the worst-case scenario, disease may be transmitted from patient to healthcare worker, or vice versa. While it is impossible to quantify the human factor, exposures clearly have a telling effect on the health of the healthcare worker and the institution.

The National Transportation Safety Board has reported a train collides with a motor vehicle between 8,000 and 9,000 times per year. As amazing as that sounds, compare it with a more astonishing statistic: 800,000 needlesticks to healthcare workers were estimated to occur in one year. The problem is further compounded by the fact that a *much larger number* of needlesticks, other sharps injuries, blood sprays, and splashes were *not* reported. Since most needlesticks and blood exposures are preventable events, it is clear hospitals have an extraordinary opportunity to realize considerable cost savings through prevention techniques.

References/Suggested Readings

Quebbeman EJ, Telford GL, Hubbard S, et al. Risk of blood contamination and injury to operating room personnel. *Ann Surg* 1991;214:614.

Tokars JI, Bell DM, Culver DH, et al. Percutaneous injuries during surgical procedures. *JAMA* 1992;267:2899.

Jagger J, Bentley M, Juillet E. Direct cost of follow-up for percutaneous and mucocutaneous exposures to at-risk body fluids: data from two hospitals. *Advances in Exposure Prevention* 1998;3(3):1.

Tereskerz PM, Jagger J. Occupationally acquired HIV: The vulnerability of healthcare workers under workers' compensation laws. *Advances in Exposure Prevention* 1998;3(3):28.

Notes

CHAPTER 3

Causes of Sharps Injuries and Exposures to Blood

The Unique Surgical Environment

The operating room has special characteristics that increase the likelihood of accidents. Workers use and pass sharp instruments contaminated with blood countless times. Additionally, the work space is confined and movement is restricted. Furthermore, although visibility of the operative site with laparoscopic surgery may be excellent on the TV monitor, visibility of the operative field for some team members may be poor during open surgery. Moreover, there is often a need for speed, and surgical team members may find themselves operating under the added stress of anxiety, fatigue, frustration, and occasionally even anger. Construction workers using dangerous power tools can stop to deal with these kinds of physical and emotional problems or even decide to quit and return the next day when conditions are safer. The surgical team, however, must continue until the procedure is completed, regardless of adverse conditions.

Another factor unique to the surgical environment is that exposures to blood often occur without the knowledge of the exposed worker until the gloves are removed at the end of the procedure, thereby prolonging the area and duration of exposure. The fingers, in particular, may frequently be the site of minor skin breaks or lacerations. These factors increase the risk of infection with bloodborne pathogens when blood comes in contact with nonintact skin, especially in the presence of high viral load.

25

Which Devices Cause Injuries?

The vast majority of hospital-based sharps injuries occur in the operating room, and most of these are from scalpel and suture-needle injuries. Because the most frequently used sharp devices during surgical procedures are suture needles and scalpels, it is not surprising these devices are responsible for the majority of glove perforations and sharps injuries. It should be kept in mind, however, that many other commonly used devices have caused percutaneous injuries and glove perforations leading to exposure to blood, including the following:

- Wire sutures
- Hollow injection needles
- Guide wires
- Stylets
- Drain trocars
- Laparoscopic trocars
- Orthopedic drill bits, screws, pins, wires, and saws
- Urethral suspension needles
- Needle point cautery tips
- Micro-scissors and other sharp pointed scissors
- Sharp pointed retractors (such as Gelpi, Wheatlander, rakes, etc.)
- Skin hooks
- Penetrating towel clips
- Tenaculi
- Thyroid clamps
- Broken glass instruments and medication vials
- Syringes (Safety syringes, commonly used for phlebotomy and injection in other hospital locations to reduce the risk of needlesticks, should be stocked in the surgical suite as well.)

When Do Injuries Occur?

Suture needle injuries often occur during the following frequently performed maneuvers:

- Mounting in needle holder
- Repositioning in needle holder
- Passing hand-to-hand between team members

- Suturing
    - Using fingers as backstop or to guide needle
    - Hand-holding tissue during suturing
    - Sewing toward fingers of surgeon or assistant
    - Protecting adjacent structures by hand of surgeon or assistant
- Manual tissue retraction or wound exposure
- Tying with needle attached
- Leaving needle on field while tying
- Holding needle in hand or needle holder while tying
- Before and after using on the field
    - Leaving needle on field contacts worker's hand
    - Dropping on worker's foot
    - Reaching for device sliding off drapes
- Placing in disposal
    - Poorly designed container
    - Overfilled container
    - Improperly positioned container
    - Poor choice of container (opening too small)

Scalpel blade injuries often occur during the following frequently performed maneuvers:
- Assembling and disassembling
- Hand-to-hand passing between team members
- During cutting
    - Using fingers as backstop
    - Hand-holding tissue during cutting
    - Cutting toward fingers of surgeon or assistant
    - Protecting adjacent structures by hand of surgeon or assistant
- Manual tissue retraction or wound exposure
- Before and after using on the field
    - Leaving scalpel on field contacts worker's hand
    - Dropping on worker's foot
    - Reaching for device sliding off drapes
- Placing in disposal
    - Overfilled container
    - Improperly positioned container

—Poor choice of container (opening too small)

During cesarean section, before the baby is delivered and placed on the field for suctioning of the nasopharynx, care is taken to remove scalpels and cautery devices from the field to prevent injury to the baby. The same care should be exercised to prevent injury to personnel. All sharps should have a designated safe location (Neutral Zone) during passing and between uses.

All Invasive Procedures are Hazardous

Some risk factors identified with increased injury and exposure rates are listed as follows:

- Procedures of prolonged duration
- Procedures associated with increased blood loss
- Many personnel in confined space

Certain surgical procedures have more than one risk factor. Orthopedic and trauma procedures, for example, are often prolonged and have increased blood loss. Cesarean sections, however, are of short duration but associated with the risk factor of increased blood loss. Abdominal and vaginal hysterectomies are usually of short duration, often with minimal blood loss, but surprisingly the injury and blood exposure rates during hysterectomy are high.

While the risk factors listed above may be helpful in understanding the causes of sharps injuries, there are two important lessons to be learned: all procedures that utilize sharps, regardless of hierarchy of risk, must be viewed as hazardous. Standard precautions must be used during all invasive procedures.

Who Is Injured or Exposed to Blood?

Surgeons are most often injured by suture needles; nurses and scrub personnel are more often injured by scalpels and other sharp devices. Circulators are not uncommonly called to participate in tasks that result in *unanticipated* exposures, including splashes of blood to the eyes because there may not have been ample time to run for equipment. Therefore, all personnel in the room should wear effective barriers appropriate to the task and anticipated degree of exposure to protect the eyes and skin (see chapter 5).

Who Injures Whom?

In one study, 33% of suturing injuries were inflicted on another worker by the person using the needle. Approximately 25% of suture needle injuries occurred during transfer between personnel. Of scalpel blade injuries, 39% were self-inflicted, while 61% were inflicted by the user of the device on assistants. The majority of scalpel injuries occurred during transfer between personnel. Strategic interventions that address these injury patterns are found in chapters 6, 7, 8, and 9.

What Are the Common Injury Sites?

Sites of scalpel and suture needle injuries are most commonly the thumb and index finger of the nondominant hand, and then in descending order the middle finger, other fingers, and palm and back of the hand. These injury sites are not unexpected, as the nondominant hand is often used to reposition or reach for needles, hold tissue being cut or sutured, or used as a retractor to protect adjacent viscera during cutting or suturing. "No-touch" techniques and other appropriate strategies that address these behavior patterns are discussed in chapters 6, 7, 8, and 9.

References/Suggested Readings

Jagger J, Blackwell B, Fowler M, Carter K, Funderburk S, Bradshaw E, Swapp J. Percutaneous injury surveillance in a 58-hospital network. *Tenth international conference on AIDS*, Yokohama, Japan, 8/9/94.

Jagger J, Balon M. Suture needle and scalpel blade injuries: frequent but underreported. *Advances in Exposure Prevention* 1995;1:1–8

Tokars JI, Bell DM, Culver DH, et al. Percutaneous injuries during surgical procedures. *JAMA* 1992;267:2889–2904.

Jagger J, Bentley M, Tereskerz P. A study of patterns and prevention of blood exposures in OR personnel. *AORNJ* 1998;67:979-996.

Notes

_____

_____

_____

_____

_____

_____

_____

What are the most common causes of sharps injuries at this surgical worksite?

suture needles _____

scalpels _____

wires _____

injection needles _____

sharp pointed scissors _____

other _____

Which procedures are most often associated with injury?

obstetrics/gynecology _____

orthopedics _____

general surgery/trauma _____

cardiovascular/thoracic _____

other _____

Which personnel most often experience exposure to blood?

surgeons _____

surgical assistants _____

scrub persons _____

circulators _____

Precautions for the Surgical Team

CHAPTER 4

General Prevention Strategies

Assuring Adequate Protection

Operating room professionals are known for going the extra mile to protect the patient, inconveniencing themselves if necessary. They should, however, spend sufficient time and effort to protect themselves. Although OSHA regulations require (hospital) employers to provide "adequate" personal protective equipment for all workers, it is appropriate for O.R. professionals to personally assume a share of the responsibility for their own protection.

The range of personal protective equipment purchased by an institution should take into account the special needs of individuals. One size or one type of device may not fit all. If currently stocked protective wear at a facility does not fill the needs of every worker and training in the correct application of an item (see chapter 5) does not solve the problem, additional equipment must be purchased. Clearly, this cannot happen unless individual needs and concerns are voiced.

Assuming Personal Responsibility

Safety in the operating room demands daily attention and maintenance. Reject the prevalent false notion that "some things will never change"—everything does. Develop a *bias for action*. Cultivate the habit of focusing simultaneously on patient safety and occupational safety throughout every procedure. Constantly observe, analyze, learn, communicate, and teach. Be a mentor to new staff members with respect to appropriate occupational safety measures just as you would with good and appropriate patient care.

Seizing Educational Opportunities

Operating room professionals may derive great benefit from observing and documenting *near exposures* as well as exposures. Take the time to think about what almost happened or what could have happened. Take advantage of these "near-misses" for they are priceless learning opportunities; discuss them at department meetings and in-services. Use the format of brainstorming, an important component of the continuous quality improvement process, to identify risk-reduction strategies.

Safety Equipment and Techniques

The methods for effectively choosing and employing specific safety procedures and techniques are fully discussed in subsequent chapters. A growing number of safety devices and techniques have shown significant results, including blunt suture needles (see chapter 7), a surgical suturing assist device to avoid manual handling of needles, a "no-touch" technique during wound closure, and double-gloving (see chapter 5). (Also see Appendix A, Safety Checklist for Operating and Delivery Rooms, designed for posting in each room.)

Safety Syringes, IV Catheters, Lancets

Hollow-bore needlesticks associated with venous access procedures and injuries from lancets may be significantly reduced by choosing appropriate equipment. A variety of intravenous catheters, phlebotomy devices, and lancets are available with features that can protect care givers by shielding or retracting the needle or lancet after use.

Needleless Intravenous Connection Systems

Surgical patients commonly require solutions and medications "piggybacked" into primary IV lines. Blood, seen or unseen, may back up into IV lines, making punctures by needles removed from IV connections a bloodborne pathogen hazard. Cases of occupational transmission of HIV, hepatitis, and tuberculosis by this mechanism have been documented. Needleless IV connection systems with valves or plug-in or twist locking mechanisms may significantly reduce the hazard of needlesticks for surgical, obstetrical, and anesthesia personnel.

Blood Collection Tubes

Injecting blood through collection tube stoppers using an exposed needle should be avoided. Instead, shielded vacuum tubes or shielded phlebotomy syringes may be used. Plastic blood collection tubes and capillary tubes are preferable to glass to avoid breakage and the creation of sharp edges, which may cause injuries.

Disposal of Blood, Body Fluids and Tissue

Disposal of large volumes of blood and body fluids (i.e., suction canister contents) and tissue may be managed most efficiently using engineering controls such as encapsulation/solidification agents. The alternative, which is direct disposal by personnel who must be fully dressed with effective protective equipment, does not eliminate the risk of exposure through spills, splashes or aerosols.

Gloving for Venous Access Procedures

Gloves are appropriate for procedures involving the use of needles, IV catheters, or other sharp devices as gloves have been shown to reduce the volume of blood contamination during needlestick injury.

Review the following General Safety Checklist and add to it in the space provided at the end of the chapter to meet personal needs.

General Safety Checklist

Absolute prerequisites:

❏ Complete the hepatitis B vaccination series

❏ Use Standard Precautions with all patients

Personal protective equipment—appropriate choices:

❏ Wear fluid-resistant head wear where appropriate.

❏ Use adequate eye and face protection.

❏ Use appropriate neck protection. Consider recently shaved skin as nonintact.

❏ Wear fluid-resistant or fluid-impervious gowns as appropriate to expected exposure risk.

❏ Choose gloves appropriately (see double-gloving, below).

❏ Wear appropriate footwear or shoe covers.

Personal protective equipment—appropriate use:
- ❏ Remove gloves carefully to avoid blood splatter.
- ❏ Wash hands with antiseptic soap after removing gloves.
- ❏ Remove eye protection last.
- ❏ Remove contaminated personal protective equipment before leaving the room.
- ❏ Carefully remove and discard mask following every procedure.

Safety techniques:
- ❏ Wear gloves when handling surgical specimens.
- ❏ Wear eye protection if container is opened or splashing is anticipated.
- ❏ Apply dressings and handle drains or packs with clean gloves.
- ❏ Avoid touching any surface with contaminated gloves.
- ❏ Avoid touching existing contaminated surfaces.

Safety strategies:
- ❏ Have extra personal protective equipment readily available should replacement be needed.
- ❏ Position sharps disposal containers at point of use.
- ❏ Have a plan for sharps management.
- ❏ Make sure all team members know the plan.
- ❏ Modify the plan as needed.
- ❏ Focus attention on sharps in use; be aware and alert.
- ❏ Alert other O.R. team members to possible hazards.
- ❏ Discourage unauthorized entry into the room.
- ❏ Keep extraneous conversation to a minimum.
- ❏ Store a tube of blood pre-operatively on all surgical patients to be held in the laboratory for possible HIV testing should an exposure occur.
- ❏ A signed consent for HIV testing, in case of an exposure, should be obtained pre-operatively to avoid delay in post-exposure follow-up.

Personal preparation:

❏ Prepare your body and mind to function effectively and efficiently.

❏ Get enough sleep before surgery. If you are working a long shift on obstetrics or trauma service, nap if and when you can.

❏ Avoid caffeine, which increases hand tremor.

❏ Avoid alcohol or other substances that impair perception, judgment, or reflexes.

❏ Promote general good health. Exercise regularly and have an annual physical.

❏ Avoid behaviors that increase nonoccupational risk of exposure to bloodborne viruses, such as unsafe sex.

References/Suggested Readings

Mast ST, Woolwine JD, Gerberding JL. Efficacy of gloves in reducing blood volumes transferred during simulated needlestick injury. *J Infect Dis* 1993;168:1589.

Trepanier CA, Lessard MR, Brochu JG, et al. Risk of cross infection related to the multiple use of disposable syringes. *Can J Anaesth* 1990;37:156.

Notes

Hazards identified: _____

_____

_____

_____

_____

_____

_____

Planned changes: _____

_____

_____

_____

_____

_____

_____

_____

Add to the checklist in this chapter as necessary: _____

_____

_____

_____

_____

_____

CHAPTER 5

Choices of Effective Personal Protective Equipment (PPE)

Why We Need "Advanced" Precautions

OSHA mandates "adequate" protection be used, but what is adequate? In patients with acute or chronic active hepatitis, 1 milliliter of blood may contain 1 million to 1 billion viral particles. A single droplet of blood, especially in the eye, could represent a significant exposure. Additionally, the O.R. professional's skin, especially the hands, may not be an intact barrier to viral penetration on any given day. Allergic rashes, shearing injuries from suture tying, and weekend sports or other activities may cause unapparent breaks in the skin. Personal protective equipment should be chosen with these factors in mind. The inability to identify all patients infected with bloodborne pathogens reinforces the need for *effective* protection with all patients.

Headwear

Headwear should provide coverage appropriate for use in an invasive surgical procedure. Choose protective caps or hoods that effectively repel blood and body fluids. Always read label information on the box to see if it is intended to repel fluids. If no information is given, hold the apparel over the scrub sink, have a co-worker gently pour some water into it, and see what happens. There is nothing wrong with a cap being a fashion statement as long as its primary protective function is fulfilled.

Neckwear

Covering the neck may be an appropriate additional precaution in cases where the patient is a known carrier of bloodborne pathogens. Recently shaved skin may be regarded as nonintact. Options would be to use face shields with integrated neck protection, neck cowling, or a hooded face shield.

Eye and Face Protection

In a surveillance study of occupational blood exposures in the operating rooms at six hospitals, health care workers' eyes were identified as being the most vulnerable location for serious blood exposures and, while surgeons were exposed more than twice as often as nurses, circulating nurses had nearly the same number of eye exposures as scrub persons. These findings indicate a need for uniform use of effective eye protection by all OR personnel. Given the importance of effective protection of the mucous membranes of the eyes, nose, and mouth, choose from the following options. Try to use the device with the best coverage and make sure you can work with it.

Face Shields

Disposable plastic face shields worn over a mask provide excellent protection for the eyes, nose, and mouth. These take up little space and can be stocked at every scrub sink. Be aware stocks may be depleted by Monday morning and make it a point to designate responsibility for daily restocking. Face shields help eliminate the problem of gaps around the edges of most other types of eye wear, and the foam brow band provides a seal at the forehead to prevent blood from running into the eyes from above. This is usually sufficient except in cases of massive blood exposures (see space suits, below). There is a certain amount of glare and shimmy with face shields that reduces visibility slightly, and they render the wearer's voice slightly difficult to hear but not enough to matter with most procedures. A circulator may easily apply a face shield to a person who is already scrubbed and has forgotten to don one. However, if the use of a loupe or other magnifier is required, face shields may not be practical.

To prevent face shields from fogging:

❑ Choose an anti-fog mask. Ensure the metal memory strip in the top of the mask matches the contour of the face and the *top tie* is snug. *Do this just prior to the surgical scrub as the proper fit may be hard to reestablish if the mask is pulled down and replaced.*

❑ Prevent fogging due to perspiration by keeping the room cool.

❑ Try different brands of face shields if necessary.

Goggles/Special Eyeglasses

If you cannot use a face shield, try goggles or eyeglasses with top and side protection. Prescription glasses with these features are available.

Mask/Shield Combinations

Face masks with an integrated clear plastic eye shield are another reasonably effective option. Be aware, however, if major blood exposure is anticipated, splashes over the top of the shield may occur, as is the case with eyeglasses.

As with face shields, to prevent fogging:

❑ Ensure the metal memory strip in the top of the mask matches the contour of the face and the top tie is snug.

❑ Keep the room cool to avoid perspiration.

"Space Suits"

Hooded face shields have become popular for orthopedic procedures with good reason. Blood splatters and bone chips created by power tools present a special hazard. Potential disadvantages with this type of equipment are difficulty hearing or being heard and the possibility of overheating. Future engineering refinements may address these problems. Currently, hooded shields are not ordinarily used in pelvic or abdominal surgery, but they remain an option with extremely high-risk procedures on infected patients.

Establish Failsafe Checkpoints

Once the surgical gown has been put on, effective application of eye protection may be more difficult, may cause contamination of the gown, or may be forgotten and overlooked entirely. An effective solution is to make it the responsibility of the person gowning the other team members to check for omissions and remind them to apply appropriate eye protection with the help of the circulator.

Hazardous Premature Removal of Eye Protection

Splashes of blood to the conjunctiva have occurred during removal and disposal of gloves and other contaminated items. For this reason, eye protection and masks should be worn during the *entire* procedure. *The procedure is not considered over until all biohazardous materials have been placed in appropriate bags or containers.*

Surgical Gown Selection

Select surgical gowns to match the expected degree of exposure. For procedures associated with significant blood loss and of prolonged duration, choose gowns with adequate length as well as maximum impermeability characteristics. (This is referred to in the industry as "strike through" protection.) If massive blood or fluid contamination is expected, impervious gowns should be long enough to extend below the top of knee-high shoe covers or boots. For procedures with low risk of exposure, such as ophthalmic surgery, liquid-resistant gowns may be used, providing an opportunity for cost savings.

The weak link in all surgical gowns, regardless of impervious qualities, is the glove-gown interface. The woven fabric typically used for the sleeve cuff feels comfortable but can act as a wick if blood seeps under the top of the glove during deep intra-abdominal and obstetric procedures. Until industry is able to provide gowns with an improved cuff design, this problem needs to be addressed. Options that have been suggested include the use of sleeve reinforcements, rubber bands (commercially packaged and sterilized) around the top of gloves, and putting on the first layer of gloves before the gown. The author and others at DeKalb Medical Center have found elbow-length (extended cuff) gloves to be an effective solution.

Putting On Gowns and Gloves After the Procedure Has Started

If the scrub person's gloves are contaminated with blood or body fluids, additional personnel scrubbing into the procedure should put on their own gown and gloves using appropriate sterile technique or receive them from personnel with uncontaminated gloves.

Studies on Glove Failure: The Rationale for Double-Gloving

Transmission of hepatitis B and hepatitis C from healthcare worker to patient and vice versa has occurred in the absence of breaks in technique and with apparently intact gloves. In a recent simulated glove use study, bacteriophage virus was found to migrate in a fluid medium through intact latex surgical gloves 18 to 42% of the time, depending upon glove type and manufacturer.

Latex is by nature a lattice-like material containing many microscopic clefts and tunnels that can fill with fluid. As gloves become "hydrated," a pathway may be created for the migration of pathogens. Hydration could occur internally with exposure to perspiration on the wearer's hands and externally with exposure to water, saline, and other fluids in surgical wounds. Additionally, exposure to fat in wounds has a degrading effect on gloves; hours into a prolonged procedure it is frequently noted the fingers of the gloves have actually become longer. Gloves apparently lose their integrity as a barrier long before such visible changes occur.

In a study of 3,018 gloves from 800 surgical procedures, it was shown the likelihood of barrier loss increased with the length of the procedure. Glove failure rates for procedures lasting less than one hour were 13%, one to three hours, 27%, three to five hours, 47%, and over five hours, 58%.

Studies have shown unused surgical gloves may leak up to 4% of the time. In fact, 1.5% and 4% have been designated as "acceptable" leak rates by regulatory agencies for surgical and examination gloves, respectively. In a recent study, defects were found in 1.4% of 210 unused surgical gloves, and in 35% of 230 gloves tested post-operatively. Numerous studies comparing single- and double-gloving show significant reduction of blood contamination of the hands when they are double-gloved. In one such study, out of 45 procedures visible blood on the surgeon's hands was noted in 38% of single-gloved procedures whereas in double-gloved procedures the rate was 2%.

The evidence suggests a single layer of gloves provides less than adequate protection and routine double-gloving appears to be a more appropriate practice. In further support of double-gloving, it is believed that important factors determining cross-infection with viral pathogens such as HIV and hepatitis are the volume of blood entering the injury site and the viral titer in the blood. If a needle contaminated with blood passes through two layers of gloves versus one layer, more blood will be stripped off the needle before it penetrates the skin, and the infection risk might be lower.

Gloving Options

The question of which combination of gloves to use when double-gloving has been the subject of some discussion. There is clearly no "right" answer, but the author has found it extremely effective to wear a medium-weight glove under a regular-weight glove, both of the same size normally worn. Others have recommended the use of different sizes of gloves for the inner and outer layer. A recent evaluation of different brands of gloves at DeKalb Medical Center revealed even the *same sizes* of gloves can actually vary by manufacturer. It pays to experiment with different glove combinations to suit individual needs.

For gynecologic surgery and operative obstetrics, the author found two pair of heavyweight (orthopedic) gloves or even two pair of medium-weight gloves uncomfortable with which to work. (Remember the author routinely operates with minimal or no sharps.) Orthopedists, however, may prefer two layers of heavyweight gloves for extra protection during procedures where gloves are subjected to increased stress. Again, experimentation to suit individual needs is required.

Double-gloving is efficient and cost-effective after the procedure is over. The outer gloves are removed and the clean inner gloves may be used to apply the wound dressing and perform other cleanup activities.

Routinely Changing Gloves and Alarm Systems

During prolonged procedures, some have advocated changing gloves every one to two hours to compensate for glove leakage over time. An additional or alternative option might be the use of glove combinations that reveal a breach in the outer layer by a visible color change.

Another possible option would be the use of an electronic device designed to trigger an alarm, alerting the wearer of a fluid breach in the gloves or gown. While such devices would not prevent an exposure, they would limit the area of exposure and the amount of exposure time by notifying the wearer to promptly change gloves and disinfect the hands. In patients with known bloodborne pathogens, these additional precautions may be appropriate. Well-planned product evaluation should be used to determine the effectiveness and cost-effectiveness of the routine use of such devices (see chapter 17, product evaluation).

Impervious Gloves and Glove Liners

The use of gloves and glove liners made of Kevlar, leather, steel mesh, and similar materials may be appropriate in orthopedic and trauma-related procedures where sharp, tearing foreign bodies are often encountered. Many of these glove materials may not, however, provide maximum protection against needle punctures. Varying degrees of interference with tactile sensation is the tradeoff when using such products, and potential users must take this into account.

Safe Removal of Gloves

Carefully remove gloves one layer at a time to avoid splashes to personnel. Never "shoot" gloves into the trash container; this dangerous practice has caused exposures to the eyes of healthcare workers standing nearby. Removing gloves one layer at a time provides important information as to whether your protective equipment was effective. Inspect each layer for the presence of blood or perforations, and inspect the hands to be sure an exposure has not occurred. If the gown sleeves are contaminated with blood, and the outer layer of gloves cannot be removed without rolling down the inner layer, then the gown should be removed first, followed by both layers of gloves, simultaneously, to avoid contamination of the hands. Wash hands after every procedure following removal of gloves; this is an OSHA requirement regardless of the number of gloves worn. Pulling on retractors, bones, and other abrasive materials stresses gloves maximally. Even multiple layers of gloves can fail depending upon the stresses to which they were subjected.

Latex Allergy

A growing danger for patients, latex allergy is an occupational health hazard for healthcare workers as well. OSHA regulations require employers to provide gloves with which operating room professionals may safely work. Nonlatex alternative gloves should be stocked at all work sites for workers who are allergic to latex. Report any rash on the hands to allow evaluation for possible latex allergy, as breaks in the skin can serve as portals of entry for bloodborne pathogens.

Footwear/Shoe Covers

Fluid-resistant disposable shoe covers are helpful in preventing exposures. Trauma boots (knee-high shoe covers) are appropriate for obstetrical procedures, other procedures associated with large volumes of blood and body fluids and the use of large volumes of irrigation fluids. Remove shoe covers before taking off gloves and before leaving the room.

Surgical Drape Selection

As is the case with all surgical attire, drapes should be selected to match the expected degree of exposure. While the advantages of impervious drapes are obvious, they cause more runoff. Drapes with an integrated waterproof pouch, therefore, are appropriate for cesarean section, vaginal delivery, hysteroscopy, arthroscopy, and similar procedures utilizing large volumes of irrigation fluid. Drapes with pouches provide the following advantages:

- Protection of personnel against exposure
- Prevention of gross contamination of the room
- Cost savings through shortening room turnover time

References/Suggested Readings

Arena B, Maffulu N, Vocaturo I, et al. Incidence of glove perforation during cesarean section. *Ann Chir Gynaecol* 1991;80:387–390.

Chapman S, Duff P. Frequency of glove perforations and subsequent blood contact in association with selected obstetric surgical procedures. *Am J Obstet Gynecol* 1992;168:1354–1357.

Cohn GM, Seifer DB. Blood exposure in single versus double gloving during pelvic surgery. *Am J Obstet Gynecol* 1990;162:715–717.

Esteban JI, Gomez J, Martell M, et al. Transmission of hepatitis C virus by a cardiac surgeon. *NEJM* 1996;334:555–560.

Fay MF, Dooher D. Surgical gloves—measuring cost and barrier effectiveness. *AORN J* 1990;55:1500–1516.

Harpaz R, Von Seidlein L, Averhoff FM, et al. Transmission of Hepatitis B virus to multiple patients from a surgeon without evidence of inadequate infection control. *NEJM* 1996;334:549– 554.

Howard R, Bennett NT. Quantity of blood inoculation in a needlestick injury from suture needles. *J Am Coll Surg* 1994;178:107–110.

Jagger J, Bentley M, Tereskerz P. A study of patterns and prevention of blood exposures in OR personnel. *AORNJ* 1998;67:979-96.

Rabussay D. Infection control and latex glove failure. *Medical Electronics* 1997; (June):46–48.

Russel TR, Roque FF, Miller FA. New detection of the leaky glove. *Arch Surg* 1996;93:245.

Shikita T, Karasawa T, Abe K, et al. Hepatitis B antigen and infectivity of hepatitis B virus. *J Infect Dis* 1997;136:571.

Notes

Hazards identified: _____

_____

_____

_____

_____

_____

_____

_____

_____

_____

Planned changes: _____

_____

_____

_____

_____

_____

_____

_____

_____

_____

_____

_____

_____

CHAPTER 6

Choices of Safer Sharps and Other Technology

It is helpful to get into the habit of thinking of sharps and related technology in a way that assigns a hierarchy of risk to them in terms of injury or glove puncture (see table 6.1). This is similar to the default setting on your computer and will facilitate automatically choosing the safest device. Try the following mental exercise.

First, imagine you are about to perform or participate in a procedure on a patient with AIDS and a high viral load and resistance to two commonly used antiretroviral drugs. The patient was started on a third drug three months ago, raising the possibility of additional cross-resistance. The procedure will last for several hours and, typical of surgical procedures in general, will require cutting, hemostasis, retraction, and transfer of sharps between surgical team members. At any given stage of the procedure, would you ask for a scalpel when a scissor would do just as well? Would you use a scissor with sharp pointed tips when one with blunt tips would do just as well? Develop a mental picture of commonly used sharps. Devices that look sharp, pointy, and dangerous *are* dangerous.

Next, imagine you are about to perform or participate in a procedure on a patient who had a flu-like illness three weeks ago or a blood transfusion recently, or does not consistently practice safe sex and whose business requires international travel. This patient looks "low risk" and may be, but how do you know? If the scissor worked as well as the scalpel for the AIDS patient and the performance of the procedure was not compromised, why not follow the same protocol here? Taking it one step further, why not with *all* patients?

Using the least dangerous device that will efficiently accomplish the procedure is an example of the concept of *Advanced Precautions.* For example, Standard Precautions simply require you wear gloves with both patients. You would likely be wearing two pair of gloves with the first (AIDS) patient, but why not with the second patient (and all patients) as well? The choices of devices selected for use during surgical procedures may significantly influence rates of injuries and exposures to blood. Because scalpel blades with pointed tips (#11 blades) cause deeper wounds than those with rounded tips, rounded blades should be chosen whenever possible.

While scalpel blades perform best when very sharp, this is not necessarily the case with suture needles. Prime examples of devices that protect the surgical team without sacrificing patient safety or performance are blunt suture needles and blunt retractors. An additional advantage of selecting blunted devices is that they may protect patients from injury or increased blood loss.

FUNCTION	SAFER	NOT AS SAFE	LEAST SAFE
Cutting	scissors, blunt tip cautery	scissors, sharp tip	scalpel
Hemostasis	blunt suture staples cautery	sharp suture	wire suture
Retraction	blunt retractor	sharp retractor	fingers or hands
Sharps transfer	Neutral Zone		hand-to-hand
PPE	double gloves	single gloves	no gloves

Table 6.1. Hazard reduction and choice of technology

Sharps and technology designed to safely manage them may be divided into two categories: those that do not and those that do require the user to activate the safety feature.

Devices That Do Not Require User Activation

Devices with *passive safety features* have "built-in" protection. Although this may make them intrinsically safer than devices that must be user-activated, it does *not* mean, however, that training in their proper use is not required. Accordingly, when using blunt-tipped suture needles, attention to proper technique is a basic requirement (see chapter 7).

Examples:
- Blunt-tipped suture needles
- Blunted retractors
- Scissor or cautery (vs. scalpel) for cutting
- Staplers (vs. sutures) for skin closure, bowel anastomosis, and hemostasis
- Synthetic (vs. wire) sutures
- Vascular clips (vs. sutures) for small bleeders deep in the pelvis
- Disposable scalpels (to avoid injuries during assembly and disassembly)

Devices That Require User Activation

This category of devices requires the user to activate the safety feature. In most cases, this means more training and in-servicing may be required when compared to devices with passive safety features.

Examples:
- Neutral Zone (Safe Zone): trays, basins, mats, Mayo stand, etc., for passing sharps (The user chooses and positions the device. See chapter 8 for optimal use.)
- Scalpels with shields or retracting blades
- Scalpel handles and devices that release blades without the need for using fingers
- Devices for parking and repositioning suture needles without using fingers
- Needle holders designed to shield the needle point while passing or tying
- Second layer of latex gloves (See chapter 5 for selection criteria, sizes, and configurations.)

References/Suggested Readings

MMWR 1997; 46:25–29. Centers for Disease Control and Prevention. Evaluation of blunt suture needles in preventing percutaneous injuries among health-care workers during gynecological surgical procedures—New York City, March 1993–June 1994.

Surgical Clinics of North America: Prevention of Transmission of Bloodborne Pathogens. Rhodes RS, Bell DM, eds. 75:6 Dec. 1995.

Notes

Hazards identified: _____

_____

_____

_____

_____

_____

_____

_____

Planned changes:

- ❑ Increased use of alternatives to scalpel.
- ❑ Increased use of blunt suture needles.
- ❑ Use of blunt retractors, nonpenetrating towel clips.
- ❑ Other

_____

_____

_____

_____

_____

_____

_____

_____

_____

CHAPTER 7

Blunt Alternatives to Sharps

Blunt-Tipped Suture Needles

Blunt-tipped suture needles are a prime example of engineering controls that prevent injury. In a number of studies from the United Kingdom, blunt needles were found to significantly reduce the rate of percutaneous injuries and/or glove perforations. A recent multicenter study conducted by the CDC in the northeastern United States found blunt needles caused no percutaneous injuries, reduced the incidence of blood contacts resulting from glove perforations eightfold, and were well accepted by the surgeons once they were educated in their use. In a surveillance study of occupational blood exposures in the operating rooms at six hospitals, the authors found that suture needle injuries were the predominant cause of injury in the OR, estimating that use of blunt suture needles alone could reduce total injuries in the OR by 30%. Richard Smith, a British surgeon and author who uses blunt needles extensively, once made the following bold but appropriate statement: "It is unethical to use sharp needles where blunt needles may be successfully used because of the reduced rate of injury with blunt needles."

Indications and Applications

Since Universal Precautions and Standard Precautions dictate the blood of all patients must be considered as infectious, the use of blunt suture needles is appropriate with all patients, regardless of their perceived risk status. Modern blunt suture needles may be successfully used somewhere during most general surgical, trauma, thoracic, gynecologic, and obstetric procedures, and are extremely advantageous for incisional closure (all layers except skin). Surgeons in almost all sub-specialties, therefore, may take advantage of this safer technology.

Blunt suture needles cannot ordinarily be used for microsurgery, or for subcuticular closure as subcuticular tissue is too dense for easy penetration. For these indications and for densely scarred fascia, sharp suture needles remain an appropriate choice. Alternatively, skin closure may be safely performed with staples to complete a "no sharps" closure. (It should be kept in mind, however, staples are considered a "sharp," especially during and after removal.) Episiotomy and perineal or vaginal laceration repair may be easily accomplished using suture needles with minimally blunt points (see chapter 12).

Cost and Availability

When initially introduced, modern blunt sutures were considerably more expensive than traditional sharp sutures, and at publication, the additional cost gap was narrowing. Like other commodities, increased usage and volume of sales of blunt needles will likely lead to more or less equivalent pricing to sharp needles. The range of suture materials available with blunt needles continues to expand as surgeons and other O.R. professionals provide feedback to the industry (see table 7.1).

Patient Safety

When blunt sutures are *selected appropriately* and a few simple techniques are followed, they appear to cause no more trauma to tissue than sharp needles and may actually be less traumatic. An interesting comparison is the Sprotte needle used for spinal anesthesia. Designed with a somewhat blunted tip to separate the fibers of the dura rather than cut through it, this blunt needle causes less leakage of cerebrospinal fluid, reducing the incidence of post-spinal headaches. The largest diameter of most suture needles, both blunt and sharp, is at the middle not the tip. Slightly to moderately blunted suture needle tips may possibly find a less traumatic path through tissue by separating fibers and sliding around small blood vessels, whereas sharp needles are more likely to lacerate them and cause bleeding. The author and others have noted less bleeding from needle exit points with blunt needles, and blood loss was not found to be increased in the large study conducted by the CDC. The use of blunt needles for decades to suture the liver and kidney illustrates the less traumatic advantage provided by blunt needle tips. Closure of peritoneal and myometrial surfaces is particularly effective because, as with the liver capsule, the tissue is less likely to be lacerated by the blunt needle.

Needle Selection: How Blunt Is Blunt?

The range of bluntness in commercially available needles varies considerably and may undergo further change as surgeons provide feedback to industry. The *least blunt* needles currently available require almost no additional conscious effort by the surgeon to penetrate tissue, while retaining most of their protective advantage. These work well for most applications, including episiotomy repair. The difference compared to a sharp needle can be almost imperceptible.

In fact, one of the author's favorite "tricks" is to ask the obstetrician or surgeon assisting him to close the fascia on the assistant's side of a Pfannenstiel incision, and then ask if the assistant realized he or she had used a blunt needle. After such a demonstration, surgeons will usually ask for a change to be made to blunt sutures on their preference cards. The least blunt needles may be used almost anywhere in abdominal and pelvic surgery, with the exception of bowel anastomosis. (A report from Scotland indicated successful use with bowel anastomosis, but the needles employed by the authors were reusable Mayo needles that had been blunted in the hospital workshop and the degree of bluntness was not described.)

When needles with an *intermediate degree of bluntness* are used, a minimally conscious effort is required to penetrate tissue such as fascia. Although perhaps not as popular as the least blunt variety, these needles may be chosen for fascial closure and for increased protection of the gloves and fingers when operating on patients with known bloodborne pathogens.

Needles that are *extremely blunt tipped* do not penetrate tissue such as fascia easily and should not be used for this purpose. Their use may be appropriate in unusual situations in pelvic and abdominal surgery where the needle absolutely must be retrieved with the fingers. If these are incorrectly chosen to suture dense tissue, such as scarred fascia, a point of diminishing return is reached. Hazard may be increased by bending or breakage of the needle, resulting in sudden unintended motion of the needle and possible injury.

In summary, the *selection criteria* for blunt suture needles should be determined primarily by the density of the tissue being sutured; another factor might be the risk status of the patient. Choose from the available menu of blunt suture needles, and match the bluntness of the tip to the suturing task. What needs to be emphasized is the full range of blunt needles all have a place in the surgical armamentarium. As the variety of blunt suture needles continues to expand, operating room professionals should avail themselves of the opportunity to evaluate various needles for specific suturing tasks, and establish optimally safe suturing protocols.

Blunt Suturing Technique

When selected and used optimally, blunt-tipped suture needles are efficacious and user- friendly. The following method has been found to yield maximum performance. The blunter the tip, the more important it is to follow these points of technique.

- Use a strong needle holder and fully activate the lock.
- Mount the needle in the mid-curve, rather than 3/4 of the way back, to prevent slippage or bending of the needle. (This is not always necessary when using minimally blunt needles.)
- Grasp and stabilize the tissue to be sutured to facilitate needle penetration.

Pitfalls and cautions include the following:

Because the less blunt the point the greater the possibility of a glove puncture, it is always advisable to *avoid manual handling* of any and all suture needles, whether blunt or sharp.

- Blunt GI needles made of thin gauge wire construction with a thin point could cause a percutaneous injury if a blow to the skin is delivered with force.
- To avoid needle breakage, thin gauge needles should not be used with dense tissue.

- Blunt needles of general closure size, especially those with minimally blunt points, could also cause a puncture if a blow to the skin is delivered with force.

- Carefully read labels on suture packs to verify blunt rather than sharp needles were pulled (see below).

Facilitating the Identification of Blunt Sutures

To avoid confusion between sharp and blunt sutures, it is important to note the current labeling practices of the major manufacturers of blunt suture needles (see also table 7.2).

- *Ethicon* blunt sutures are identified by the registered trade name *ETHIGUARD* in small print on the front of the package. At the time of publication, the word *ETHIGUARD* printed *in red type on the box* containing the suture packs was the only identifier of the *minimally blunt point* on some of the needles supplied by Ethicon.

- *Sherwood Davis & Geck* blunt sutures are identified by the registered trade name *Protect-point* in small print on the front of the package. Also found in small print at the upper left-hand corner is the description *Modified Taper Needle(s)*.

- *United States Surgical Company* blunt sutures are identified by the words *BLUNT POINT* on the opening flap on the front of the package.

Use the conversion chart (table 7.1) for ease of identification. Update the chart as more blunt sutures become available.

Labeling codes on blunt suture packages, 1998:

Ethicon

- CTB-1 (vs. CT)=blunt
- SHB (vs. SH)=blunt
- CTXB (vs. CTX)=very blunt

Sherwood Davis & Geck

- MT-12=blunt
- MT-20=blunt
- MT-25=blunt
- MT-56=very blunt
- MT-60=blunt

United States Surgical Corporation

- BGS=blunt

Table 7.1. Blunt suture conversion chart
Copyright © 1999. *Advanced Precautions for Today's O.R.*
This page may be copied without written permission.

Ethicon

- *Coated Vicryl
- *Monocril
- *PDS II
- *Prolene
- silk
- gut-chromic

Sherwood Davis & Geck

- *Dexon
- *Maxon
- *Surgilene
- chromic catgut

United States Surgical Corporation

- *Polysorb
- *Biosyn
- *Surgipro
- *Surgigut

(*Trade names)

Table 7.2. Suture materials available with blunt needles

Copyright © 1999. *Advanced Precautions for Today's O.R.*

This page may be copied without written permission.

The following steps show a safe method for separating detachable sutures from blunt and sharp needles:

1. With the dominant hand, securely grasp the needle with the needle holder near the back end (not near the needle tip) to prevent the needle from flying off during separation.

2. With the nondominant hand, grasp the suture material close to the needle.

3. With the fingers of the dominant and nondominant hands in close proximity, push with the nondominant thumb against the needle holder to separate the needle from the suture. A sudden release is avoided, preventing the loaded needle holder from swinging in an arc and causing injury.

When using swedged on sutures, either park the needle safely between uses or remove the needle from the suture before tying.

Other blunt alternatives include:
- Staples for skin closure as an alternative to sutures
- Scissors with rounded rather than pointed tips
- Nonpenetrating towel clips
- Blunted retractors in place of sharp versions
- Synthetic sutures in place of wire sutures
- Hemostatic clips vs. sutures, where appropriate
- Alternatives to scalpel for cutting tasks, such as scissors or cautery

Other examples of preferred safe technology are listed below:
- Disposable scalpels, to avoid the need for blade removal and facilitate safe disposal
- Scalpels with shielded or retractable blades
- Suturing assist devices that allow one-handed suturing to avoid manual handling of needles
- LLETZ loop for conization vs. pointed scalpel.

Especially Dangerous Devices

The use of hand-held *straight suture needles* is associated with a reported injury rate of 17%, an unnecessary risk since safer alternatives exist. Anesthesiologists, radiologists, and others who close incisions for vascular access sites should be made aware of this hazard. The use of curved needles with a needle holder or staples for skin closure are safer options.

Wire sutures are associated with high rates of percutaneous injury. There is a documented case report of probable infection of a cardiovascular surgeon with HIV during the use of wire sutures for sternal closure.

Surgeons' Preference Cards: A Failsafe Checkpoint for Safe Technology

As safer technology is adopted into routine practice, preference for blunt sutures, blunt retractors, and other safety devices should appear on the surgeon's preference card. This will help to ensure that these items are always available at the *beginning* of the procedure. If the less safe technology was pulled in error, the temptation is to use what is on the table, simply because it is already there. Wait for the safer alternative to be provided if the patient's condition permits. Reinforce good habits and lead by example.

Surgeons' and Hospitals' Feedback to Industry

Traditionally, the suture market has been driven by surgeons' requests for sharper and sharper needles. Now that the pendulum is swinging toward the inclusion of safer product options, industry needs to know exactly what surgeons want. As the need for specific variations are identified, surgeons' preferences for a wider variety of blunt tipped suture needles, and other safer devices, should be made known to company representatives so that industry may respond to our needs.

References/Suggested Readings

Bebbington MW, Treissman MJ. The use of a surgical assist device to reduce glove perforations in postdelivery vaginal repair: a randomized controlled trial. *Am J Obstet Gynec* 1996;175:862–866.

Dauleh MI, Irving AD, Townell NH. Needle prick injury to the surgeon—do we need sharp needles? *J R Coll Surg Edinb* 1994 (Oct.);39(5):310–311.

Haiduven D, Allo M. Evaluation of a one-handed surgical suturing device to reduce intraoperative needlestick injuries and glove perforations. *Infect Control Hosp Epidemiol* 1994;15:344 and 1520 (supplement).

Hartly JE, Ahmed S, Milkins R, Naylor G, Monson JRT, Lee PWR. Randomized trial of blunt-tipped versus cutting needles to reduce glove puncture during mass closure of the abdomen. *Br J Surg* 1996;83:1156–1157.

Jagger J, Bentley M, Tereskerz P. A study of patterns and prevention of blood exposures in OR personnel. *AORNJ* 1998;67:979-96.

Mingoli A, Sapienza P, et al. Influence of blunt needles on surgical glove perforation and safety for the surgeon. *Am J Surg* 1996;172:512–517.

MMWR 1997;46:25–29 Centers for Disease Control and Prevention. Evaluation of blunt suture needles in preventing percutaneous injuries among health-care workers during gynecological surgical procedures— New York City, March 1993–June 1994.

Montz FJ, Fowler JM, Farias-Eisner R, Nash TJ. Blunt needles in fascial closure. *Surg Gynecol Obstet* 1991;173(2):147–148.

Rotheram EB, Jr. Probable transmission of HIV from patient to physician during surgery. *Infect Control Hosp Epidemiol* 1994;15:349.

Wright KU, Moran CG, Briggs PJ. Glove perforation during hip arthroplasty. A randomized prospective study of a new taperpoint needle. *J Bone Joint Surg Br* 1993 (Nov); 75(6):918–920.

Notes

Hazards identified: _____

_____

_____

_____

_____

_____

Planned changes: _____

_____

_____

_____

_____

_____

Preferred suture materials: _____

_____

_____

_____

_____

Availability with blunt needles:

    yes

    no

Acceptable substitute suture material with blunt needles: _____

_____

_____

Plan: contact manufacturer to request blunt needles with preferred suture material/length

CHAPTER 8

Team Tactics and Techniques for Handling Sharps

Everyone Must Lead

Any member of the surgical team should immediately react appropriately upon perceiving a real or potential hazard. Students or new graduates, in particular, should know this is an important function and should not hesitate to point out an impending hazard. For example, "I think you forgot your eye protection," or "Let's remove that needle from the suture before you tie." Everyone, at one time or another, must assume a leadership role in hazardous work sites.

The Power of Synergy

In previous chapters we have seen how individuals can immediately and significantly reduce their occupational risk by selecting the safest personal protective equipment and sharps technology. To take exposure prevention to the next level, however, teamwork is required. The importance of team interaction and good verbal communication cannot be emphasized enough. There is, perhaps, no better example of this than appropriate use of the Neutral Zone (Safe Zone).

Transferring Sharps Safely: The Neutral Zone (Safe Zone)

One fourth of suture needle injuries and more than half of scalpel injuries occur during passing. A strategic intervention gaining in popularity is the use of a Neutral Zone (Safe Zone) in which sharps may be placed and retrieved. Various devices such as mats, trays, basins, all or part of an instrument stand, or a designated area on the field have been used as a Neutral Zone. Some work better than others, however, and some may actually be dangerous.

An example of a poor choice is the ubiquitous kidney basin: Items are hard to pick up, fingers tend to wind up inside—in close proximity to the sharp—and these basins tend to tip over. The kidney basin is well designed for holding urine and should be left for that purpose. Ideally, a device selected to serve as the neutral zone should be large enough to adequately contain the sharps used, not easily tipped over, and preferably mobile without placing fingers inside the transfer tray.

Some operating room professionals still may be reluctant to abandon tradition and use a Neutral Zone. Others, having accepted the concept as potentially beneficial, may not use it in an optimal manner. Even worse, through inappropriate use, the risk of injury may actually be increased. The following principles and guidelines are suggested for optimally safe use of the Neutral Zone. The configuration of personnel at the operating table may dictate changes or additions. Add to the following list of guidelines those specific procedures necessary for your individual needs.

General Principles of the Neutral Zone (NZ)

Purpose: To reduce the incidence of percutaneous injuries and blood exposures by reducing the incidence of hand-to-hand transfer of sharps, a common cause of injury.

Exceptions: Hand-to-hand transfer of sharps remains an appropriate option at the surgeon's discretion in situations when he or she cannot avert eyes from the field or cannot reach the NZ because of positioning or other factors.

Caution: As with any other device or protocol intended for injury prevention, improper, thoughtless, or careless use may increase rather than decrease the hazard.

Suggested Guidelines for Safe and Effective Application of the Neutral Zone

- Before the first incision or injection is made, the NZ is selected and designated by the surgeon in consultation with the person passing instruments.

- The NZ is dedicated to sharps only; all other instruments are passed hand-to-hand.

- Only one sharp is to occupy the NZ at any time.

- The scrub person announces the sharp by name when placing it in the NZ ("suture," "scalpel," etc.). Alternatively, rather than name the sharp, the scrub person may say "safe zone."

- The scrub person does not hold the NZ device but leaves it in the intended location on the field to keep fingers out of harm's way.

- The scrub person orients the sharp in the NZ so the surgeon may pick it up with the dominant hand without the need for turning or repositioning.

- The scrub person ensures suture needles are mounted and positioned optimally to avoid the need for the surgeon to reposition them in the needle holder. The Safety Checklist (see Appendix A) should indicate whether the surgeon is right- or left-handed.

- Using a team approach, the surgeon and scrub person communicate freely to determine the optimal placement of the NZ for a given procedure and at different times during the procedure. The NZ may be moved at will and by agreement to accommodate the surgeon's needs.

Avoiding Breaks in Sterility

The practice of leaving suture needles on the field should be avoided for the following reasons:

- Needle tips facing down may penetrate the drapes and increase the risk of wound infection because of staph epidermidis.

- Needle tips left facing up may result in recognized or unrecognized glove punctures and blood exposures.

Ancillary Safe Techniques for Sharps Transfer

- When hollow-bore needles are used for injection of hemostatic agents during, for example, plastic procedures, vaginal hysterectomy, myomectomy, conization, or other procedures, the needle may be left in the tissue if refilling of the syringe is required. The syringe is then disconnected and refilled and reattached to the needle. The use of a long or spinal needle maintains distance between the needle point and the fingers.

- If the NZ becomes contaminated, the point of a suture needle may be protected during passing by clamping over the tip with the needle holder. Problems with this technique include breaking off the point of the needle or having the needle fly off if the jaws of the needle holder release unexpectedly. A special needle holder has been designed with a groove along the jaws to accept the needle point and grasp the needle more securely.

- Before pulling a sharp drain trocar through an exit wound, replace the guard onto the tip using a grasping instrument rather than the fingers.

- In addition to using a neutral zone for loaded suture carriers, special devices that adhere to the drapes have been designed in which one may more safely park needles between uses.

Educational Opportunities

- Bring to the attention of the O.R. manager any hazardous behavior or near- exposures you may observe; participate in brainstorming for solutions at staff meetings and in-services.

- Voice any concerns you may have. Positive change cannot occur without documentation of problems.

- Mentor new staff in techniques and protocols for exposure prevention.

- Use and update the Safety Checklist posted in each O.R. (see Appendix A).

Lessons on Teamwork From Nature

Most people know when geese migrate in V formation, each drafts off the wing of the bird in front, with the leader expending extra energy. This obviously would not work for transcontinental migration. A lesser known fact, however, is the lead is shared. Periodically, the leader rotates back, and another bird takes the lead. Birds also stay aware of each other's relative location by vocalized call notes. As a birder, part of the pleasure I derive from seeing and hearing flocks of large migratory birds— in addition to the innate beauty of the sights and sounds—is in the functionality of how they take care of each other. With a little thought, these principles can be successfully applied to exposure prevention in the O.R.

References/Suggested Readings

Jagger J, Balon M. Suture needle and scalpel blade injuries: frequent but under reported. *Advances in Exposure Prevention* 1995;1:1–8.

Jagger J, Bentley M, Tereskerz P. A study of patterns and prevention of blood exposures in OR personnel. *AORNJ* 1998;67:979-996.

Notes

Hazards identified: _____

_____

_____

_____

_____

_____

_____

_____

Planned changes: _____

_____

_____

_____

_____

_____

_____

Preferred choice of device for Neutral Zone: _____

_____

_____

_____

_____

_____

_____

CHAPTER 9

Safe Tactics and Techniques for Assisting in Surgery

The hazard associated with assisting in surgery may be markedly reduced by anticipating the needs of the surgeon for specific devices, strategic choices of equipment, safe technique, and good communication between surgical team members. Percutaneous injuries occur before, during, and after the use of sharps; opportunities for injury prevention exist in all of these situations. A simultaneous consciousness of patient safety and healthcare worker safety should prevail throughout the procedure. More and more, healthcare workers are incorporating safety techniques as key elements of surgery, driven by concern for fellow workers. This chapter focuses on safe behavior patterns for the surgical assistant to follow when sharps are in use.

Avoidance of Unnecessary Speed and Motion

When sharps are in use on the field, there is rarely a need for excessive speed. The most technically proficient surgeons finish procedures faster than less experienced surgeons not by the use of rapid hand motion but by avoiding unnecessary and repetitive movements. Good assistants, as well, strictly avoid extraneous movement, especially when sharps are in use.

Communication

Use verbal communication to help prevent collisions between hands and sharps. When a sharp is in use, avoid anticipating motion of anyone's hands; wait for the surgeon to request sponging. *Do not assume any-thing.* Often students or new graduates, eager to help, place their hands unnecessarily near sharps in use or perform needless maneuvers. Always correct this type of dangerous behavior. Surgical assistants need to know surgeons will ask for help when it is needed.

Opening the Abdomen

Sponging when the scalpel is in use may be done in one of several safe ways. Either the surgeon states he or she will do the sponging while holding the scalpel in the other hand and the assistant will only retract his or her side of the incision, or the assistant will sponge only by re-quest of the surgeon. The use of cautery rather than scalpel inherently reduces the hazard.

Options for arming and rearming suture carriers using the no-touch technique are listed below:

- When removing suture needles from suture packs, use the needle holder rather than the fingers.

- When suturing, use a Ferris-Smith forceps or similar strong for-ceps to securely regrasp and position the needle in the needle holder.

- Use commercially available suturing assist devices in which to park and regrasp the needle.

- When loading either blunt-tipped or sharp suture needles for a left-handed surgeon, the needle may be mounted as for a right-handed surgeon, then rotated 180 degrees using the above options.

Retracting

It has been said the surgeon's hand is the best retractor. While this may be true in a functional sense, use of the assistant's hands for retract-ing should be avoided unless there is no surgical retractor to accomplish the task reasonably well.

Sponging

When the surgeon is holding a sharp, sponging should be done only on verbal request of the surgeon. Even then, there is often the option the sponge can be held on a sponge stick.

Sharps Transfer

Sharps transfer through a Neutral Zone (Safe Zone) as described in chapter 8 should be the rule, with exceptions as noted.

During laparoscopic procedures, when the surgeon requests a long, sharp-pointed instrument or hollow-bore needle, the person passing instruments may, if the surgeon desires, use both hands to safely place the tip inside the port sleeve, keeping both hands behind the tip. The handle can then be angled toward the surgeon's waiting hand. Alternatively, the surgeon or surgical assistant can perform this maneuver in a similar or modified fashion.

Steps for safe assembly and disassembly of sharps include the following:

- Assemble and disassemble sharp devices in a safe and unhurried manner. Prepare in advance whenever possible and anticipate the need for the device.

- Mount and remove scalpel blades and needles with safety devices designed for this purpose or with a hemostat—never with the fingers.

- When assembling or dismantling devices with sharp components requires the use of both hands and an opposing push-pull motion, it should be done with extreme care. If possible, both hand-held components should be placed on a stable flat surface to limit the possible plane of motion to two rather than three dimensions.

Safe techniques for recapping and disposal are listed below:

- Recapping of needles should ideally be totally avoided by direct disposal. If needles must be reused during a procedure for incremental injection, use safety-engineered recapping devices or long-handled instruments—never the fingers. Placement of the needle and the cap on a flat level surface will limit the chance of the needle tip traveling in a three-dimensional plane.

- Another option for managing needles between uses is to stick the needle into a towel rolled as a tube.

- Crossing the room with sharps in hand has resulted in injuries. Sharps disposal containers should be placed as close as possible to the point of use, preferably within arm's reach.

- An important principle to remember is to *keep both hands behind the needle*—the same as with safe phlebotomy, injection, and intravenous catheter insertion techniques.

Sharps containers should be chosen and managed as follows:

- Openings of sharps disposal containers should be large enough for the intended devices.

- Access to the opening should remain unobstructed.

- Avoid overfilling the container.

- Never reach into a sharps disposal container with fingers or instruments. Once disposed of, sharps are not to be retrieved from containers.

- Designate and understand whose responsibility it is to change containers when the full line has been reached.

Avoid "unnecessary" assisting. For example:

- Keep hands away from the incision during cutting and suturing.

- Try not to lean over the incision when suturing or cutting is to take place.

Safe Retrieval of Dropped Sharps

If a sharp starts to slip off the drapes, avoid reaching for it. If a sharp falls to the floor, the circulator should use a magnet or other appropriate instrument to retrieve it. If a bloody scalpel blade falls and sticks to the floor, avoid using the fingers in an attempt to pick it up. A scalpel blade mounted on a handle may be used to pry the stuck blade up, while a towel or inverted container is held over the blade to prevent it from flying up.

Unusual Situations

If an unusual situation arises involving a sharp, *slow down* and think about how to best handle it safely.

Checklist for Safe Assisting and Operating:

- ❏ Avoid handling needles manually.

- ❏ Never hold a scalpel, loaded needle holder, or any other sharp in the same hand simultaneously with another instrument.

❏ Scalpels, loaded needle holders, and other sharps should be held in the hand only during cutting, suturing, or other specific tasks. At all other times, sharps should be contained in a designated zone on the field.

❏ Properly employ a Neutral Zone for the safe passing of sharps (see chapter 8).

❏ Use verbal warnings to announce transfer of sharps.

❏ Before tying, either remove the needle from the suture, park the needle safely, or protect the needle point with the needle holder.

❏ Use controlled release sutures or safety devices to facilitate needle removal.

❏ Avoid finger contact with tissue being sutured or cut.

❏ Use retractors rather than manual retracting whenever possible.

❏ Avoid reflex sponging of tissue, which may not be anticipated by the surgeon, when a sharp is in use.

❏ Keep eyes on all sharps in use until they are returned to the Neutral Zone.

❏ Pass long laparoscopic instruments, such as needle tip cautery and sharp-pointed scissors, handle first and tip down.

❏ Replace the shield onto the tip of a drain trocar with an instrument, not the fingers, before pulling the trocar out of the exit wound.

❏ When the syringe needs to be refilled because you are injecting incrementally, consider leaving the needle in the tissue, removing the syringe, refilling it, and then reattaching the syringe to the needle.

Notes

Hazards identified: _____

_____

_____

_____

_____

_____

_____

_____

Planned changes: _____

_____

_____

_____

_____

_____

_____

Add to the checklist in this chapter as necessary: _____

_____

_____

_____

_____

_____

_____

_____

CHAPTER 10

Management of Surgical Smoke

Surgical Smoke as a Health Hazard

Smoke generated with thermal destruction of tissue by electrosurgical units as well as lasers is noxious and hazardous to patients and O.R. professionals alike. Surgical smoke contains toxic gases including formaldehyde, hydrogen cyanide, and benzene. It causes irritation to the eyes and upper respiratory tract and represents an occupational risk of chronic lung disease. Surgical smoke has also been shown to contain bioaerosols, including dead and live cellular material (viral DNA particles and viable bacteria). In addition to toxic gases inhaled by healthcare workers, particulate matter in surgical smoke and laser plume is small enough to pass through surgical masks and be inhaled. The American National Standards Institute (ANSI) recommends the use of smoke evacuators and high efficiency surgical masks for laser procedures. The Association of Operating Room Nurses (AORN) recommends the aspiration of smoke during all surgical procedures.

Could Viral Pathogen Transmission Occur via Inhalation?

Infection of healthcare workers with HIV via smoke inhalation has not been reported. Although airborne transmission of HIV via surgical smoke is considered a highly unlikely theoretical risk, other studies give cause for concern. Laryngeal papillomatosis with human papilloma virus DNA has been reported in a laser surgeon. In an animal study, viral DNA particles (bovine fibropapilloma virus) were recovered from laser generated smoke during vaporization of cattle warts and reinoculated (injected) back into host cattle, resulting in new lesions.

Smoke evacuation has been well integrated into vaginal laser procedures by appropriate speculum design, but work remains to be done to eliminate the hazard of smoke generated by electrosurgical units.

Options for smoke management during open procedures include:

1. Smoke generated by electrosurgical units may be aspirated at the point of origin by commercially available portable smoke evacuators designed for aspiration of laser plume. *Caution*: If a hand-held suction wand is used, care must be taken to keep the open end far enough away from small bowel to avoid accidental aspiration of bowel loops. The use of High Efficiency Particulate Air (HEPA) filters or equivalent is recommended by the National Institute for Occupational Safety and Health (NIOSH). Other filtering and cleaning processes are also available. Filters require monitoring and replacement on a regular basis and are considered a possible biohazard requiring proper disposal.

2. Room suction systems pull at a much lower rate and were designed to capture liquids rather than particles or gases. Although not as powerful as dedicated smoke evacuators, these systems may be used to remove smoke produced by cautery. The nasal tip suction should be held just above or lateral to the cautery tip (within 2 inches) for maximally effective smoke aspiration. The smoke evacuation or suction unit should be ON at all times when cautery is in use. In-line filters are necessary if room suction is used. Tubing, filters, and absorbers are considered infectious waste and must be disposed of appropriately. (For a discussion of smoke management during laparoscopic procedures, see chapter 13.)

Improved Technology Needed

The problem with both of the above options is an assistant's hand must be dedicated to the task of smoke aspiration, and this is difficult to coordinate. Technology to better address these problems is being developed and refined. One goal should be integrated combination cautery-suction units, ideally with automatic activation of the suction component when the cautery is activated. This would eliminate the need for a dedicated assistant's hand. Effective, user-friendly, and cost-effective technology is needed. Well-planned product evaluation (see chapter 17) will facilitate the purchase of appropriate equipment.

References/Suggested Readings

Ball, K. *Lasers: The perioperative challenge* (2nd ed.). 1995. St. Louis, MO: C. V. Mosby.

Garden JM, O'Banion K, Shelnitz L, et al. Papilloma virus in the vapor of carbon dioxide laser-treated verrucae. *JAMA* 1988;8:1199–1202.

Hallimo P, Naess O. Laryngeal papillomatosis with human papillomavirus DNA contracted by laser surgeon. *Eur Arch Otorhinolaryngol* 1991;248(7):425–427.

Heinsohn P, Jewett D. Exposure to blood-containing aerosols in the operating room: a preliminary study. *Am Ind Hyg Assoc J* 1993;54(8):446–453.

U.S. Department of Health and Human Services (NIOSH) Publication No. 96-128. Control of smoke from laser/electric surgical procedures. Sept 1996.

Notes

Hazards identified: _____

_____

_____

_____

_____

_____

_____

Planned changes: _____

_____

_____

_____

_____

_____

_____

Technology currently used for smoke management: _____

_____

_____

_____

_____

_____

_____

_____

CHAPTER 11

Precautions for Anesthesia Personnel

Standard Precautions

Anesthesia personnel, like all surgical personnel, are at substantial risk of exposure to blood and body fluids. Standard Precautions should be observed to significantly reduce the risk. Masks and eye protection should be worn during intubation, extubation and suctioning, and when anticipating aerosols. It is appropriate to wear gloves during intubation, extubation, suctioning, injection, and venous or arterial access procedures. Liquid barrier garments should be worn when exposure is anticipated.

Needlesticks and Needleless IV Systems

Anesthesia personnel are at significant risk of exposure to blood through the frequent use of hollow-bore needles, injection needles, intravenous and central venous cannulas, and intra-arterial catheters. Most surgical patients have at least one vascular access device inserted, and medications are often injected into intravenous tubing ports. Fluid from intravenous tubing is considered infectious. Rather than using hollow-bore needles for this purpose, needleless IV connection systems with valves or plug-in or twist-locking mechanisms should be used, thereby significantly reducing the incidence of needlesticks. Changing from a non-safety (conventional) IV catheter to a safety IV catheter has been shown to reduce accidental needlesticks by 84%. Important features of safety IV catheters are complete shielding of the needle, audible locking of the shield, and both hands staying behind the needle.

Sharps Disposal Containers

To optimize safe disposal, sharps disposal containers may be mounted on the anesthesia supply cart within arm's reach of the person administering anesthesia. Peripheral and neuraxial blocks in surgery and obstetrics are invasive procedures requiring the use of numerous sharp objects, including hollow-bore needles, stylets, and broken glass vials. An alternative to individually disposing of multiple sharps via a small container opening would be to use a sharps disposal container with an opening large enough to accommodate the entire anesthesia tray. This may reduce the risk of injury from sharps when one disposes of a tray after a procedure.

Blood Aerosols, Blood Splashes, and Eye Protection

Despite surgical drapes screening the anesthesiologist and anesthetist from the surgical field, blood and blood aerosols may frequently pass over the screen via laparoscopic ports or directly from arterial bleeders or splashes. Effective eye and face protection should be used during every procedure based on proximity of personnel to the surgical site, *including* personnel entering and leaving the room.

Anesthesia Suction Equipment

Suction tips contaminated with blood during intubation and extubation may become a source of exposure to the eyes, and may contaminate the work site. They may be safely stored during the procedure in the disposable sheath they came in or some other device designed for this purpose.

References/Suggested Readings

Berry A. Injury prevention in anesthesiology. *Surgical Clinics of North America.* 1995 (Dec)75;6:1123–1132.

Notes

Hazards identified: _____

_____

_____

_____

_____

_____

_____

Planned changes: _____

_____

_____

_____

_____

_____

Current utilization of needleless systems: _____

_____

_____

Type of sharps disposal units currently in use: _____

_____

_____

Location of sharps disposal units: _____

_____

_____

_____

Precautions for Special Situations

CHAPTER 12

Obstetrical Procedures

Vaginal Delivery: Personal Protective Equipment

Blood contact to healthcare workers' skin and mucous membranes has been observed in 25% of vaginal deliveries and 35% of cesarean sections. Large volumes of amniotic fluid contaminated with blood are commonly encountered. Maximal sterile barriers, as recommended by the CDC, should be the standard for personal protective equipment. Personal protective equipment for obstetrical procedures should include face protection with the best possible coverage, and all garments should be highly impervious to fluid strike-through. Elbow-length gloves are useful for protecting the glove-gown interface during vaginal delivery, manual removal of the placenta, and cesarean section. Knee-high boot or shoe covers are useful for protecting the lower extremities from exposures.

Fetal Scalp Electrode Application

It is advisable to wear a face shield and gloves on both hands when inserting invasive fetal monitoring devices because when the sheath is removed from the electrode wire, splatter of blood or blood-tinged amniotic fluid may occur. The same precautions apply when removing the sheath from an intrauterine pressure catheter.

Long Gloves: Donning Technique

Long gloves have sometimes been described as difficult to put on. The following technique, successfully used by the author, takes advantage of the double fold provided by the manufacturer: Rather than fully opening the gloves initially, put on the gloves in a two-step procedure. The additional cost of long gloves is balanced by exposure prevention.

Availability and Accessibility of Personal Protective Equipment

Because delivery of the fetus or sudden hemorrhage may occur rapidly and without warning, personal protective equipment should be stored at the work site, with sufficient additional supplies nearby. Monitoring to ensure sufficient inventory is essential since obstetric personnel will have to provide patient care whether personal protective equipment is available or not.

Routine Use of Episiotomy

The question of potential benefit or harm to the patient with routine episiotomy has been the subject of debate for decades. At the present time, when significant numbers of obstetrical patients may harbor HIV or hepatitis viruses, what requires no debate is that an operative procedure avoided equals a percutaneous injury prevented. Certainly, with a known infected or high-risk patient, this may weight the decision against elective episiotomy. When faced with deciding whether to perform *any* elective procedure in the presence of known bloodborne pathogens, taking time to think through the situation may prevent a significant exposure.

To illustrate this point, as an intern on the obstetrical service in 1965, I vividly remember having been assigned the management of labor and delivery for a patient with acute fulminant viral hepatitis on the verge of hepatic coma at 34 weeks gestation. Only one month into my internship, I had already experienced several suture needlesticks. Although the prevailing wisdom at that time was all patients undergoing premature delivery were to have an episiotomy, I made a conscious decision not to perform one in this case to minimize the use of sharp suture needles and the additional blood loss associated with episiotomy.

Episiotomy Repair: Blunt Suture Needle Selection

Having described the uniqueness of the surgical environment, it can be argued the delivery room is a work site with even greater challenges. Obstetrical patients may move unexpectedly during repair of an episiotomy or vaginal laceration. There is no surgical assistant provided for these procedures. The operator's hand routinely serves as a retractor during suturing, with the suture needle tip millimeters from the fingers of the nondominant hand. The surgical light may be hard to focus on the operative site, particularly with a briskly bleeding high vaginal laceration. The danger of suturing is often compounded by poor visibility of the suture needle tip due to large amounts of blood and amniotic fluid and the tendency of the vaginal walls to collapse inward. Surgical suction is not routinely provided.

Often, the room temperature is high for the comfort of the patient and protection of the newborn, resulting in decreased visibility for the operator from perspiration and fogging of protective equipment worn over the face. Family members and other visitors provide unexpected noise and distractions. The operator may be fatigued due to lack of sleep, with resultant diminished hand-eye coordination. He or she may be stressed and distracted by concern for the condition of the parturient or the newborn.

Under these kinds of adverse conditions, the routine use of blunt-tipped suture needles provides a major opportunity to reduce the chance of a needlestick or glove perforation. Episiotomy repair is facilitated by selecting minimally blunt suture needles and using the technique described in chapter 7.

Sharps Disposal in the Labor and Delivery Room

Contaminated injection needles and suture needles left on the delivery table have frequently caused injury to obstetricians, midwives, labor and delivery nurses, obstetrical technologists, and cleaning staff. One reasonable solution is to place a needle collection box on the table. If this strategy is chosen, it is important to designate responsibility for placing the disposal device, filling and closing it, conducting a needle count as is done in the operating room, and monitoring compliance with these procedures. If only some of the needles are placed in the box and others remain on the cluttered table, the hazard will have been increased rather than decreased.

Sharps Disposal Containers

Selection

Disposal containers must be puncture-proof and have an opening of adequate size to accept the sharps used in the workplace, ideally with a childproof mechanism that prevents reaching into the opening. The "full" line should be readily visible, indicating when it is time for the container to be replaced.

Optimal Placement

Hollow-bore venipuncture needles, injection needles, and IV catheters commonly used in labor and delivery rooms carry the greatest risk of infecting care givers with bloodborne pathogens. Safe disposal has become complicated by the fact that visitors, friends, and family members, including small children, have become part of the labor and delivery setting. If a nurse or other care giver has to cross the room to reach the sharps disposal container, the risk of puncture is increased. The container should be placed as close as possible to the bedside where venipunctures and other needle-related procedures occur, ideally within arm's reach. The care giver must be able to see and reach the opening of the container easily. Access to the opening should be unrestricted vertically and laterally, away from shelves, carts, and other obstructions.

Maintenance

A full or overfilled container instantly becomes a hazard because the care giver with a used needle in hand is then faced with the choice of crossing or leaving the room to access another container or recapping the used needle, both unsafe procedures. The labor and delivery nurses should meet with the department supervisor and infection control personnel to jointly decide on optimal safe placement of containers and designate responsibility for replacement as containers become full. The users of dangerous devices in hazardous situations can provide the most valuable input as to what the existing hazards are in any given work site. It is critically important the users—in this case the nurses who draw blood, give injections, and start intravenous infusions—be involved in the decision-making process.

Checklist for Safe Sharps Disposal

❑ Choose containers with built-in safety features, such as "see-through" (translucent) boxes with a readily apparent fill level and full line.

❑ Consider containers with self-closing lids when 3/4 filled, to prevent overfilling.

❑ Lids should allow the sharp to enter the container by gravity alone, without the need for additional manipulation.

❑ Install containers close to the point of use, ideally within arm's reach.

❑ Mount containers at a convenient height for use and service, in plain sight and free from obstructions.

❑ Do not leave containers free-standing on the floor or on their side.

❑ Do not shake containers to avoid aerosolization, spillage or protrusion of sharps.

❑ Schedule staff training and education for proper use of containers.

❑ Assign responsibility for maintenance and service of containers.

Cesarean Section

As with vaginal delivery, the use of maximum eye and face protection, elbow-length gloves, and blunt-tipped suture needles for all layers except the skin are appropriate and effective for avoiding exposures to blood and percutaneous injuries. Cautery may be used to open the abdomen after the initial skin incision. Cutting cautery at a setting of 70 watts may be used to open the skin in patients harboring known bloodborne pathogens; some would argue the cosmetic result with a low transverse incision is satisfactory. The scalpel is used for incising the uterus to avoid thermal injury to the baby from cautery.

Collection of Umbilical Cord Blood Samples

When cord blood is required for diagnostic studies, it may be collected with a needleless syringe from a cup, and passed off the sterile field where unstopped collection tubes may be filled. The use of hollow-bore needles on the operative field during cesarean section is best avoided because of the rapid motion by more than one person occurring at the operative site. Cord pH and acid-base studies may be more safely obtained by clamping and cutting a segment of cord of sufficient length and handing it off the field to personnel who may then draw blood on a flat stable surface away from the busy operative site.

Newborn Circumcision

Personnel performing newborn circumcision often neglect to use eye and face protection. Bloody urine may contact the eyes, nose, or mouth, resulting in the need for post-exposure management and prophylaxis. Although the risk of infection with HIV is low, it is not nonexistent, and the risk of infection with hepatitis is significant. Exposures in this setting are easily preventable in a cost-effective manner by wearing a fluid shield face mask or visor.

A disposable scalpel is the preferred choice of scalpel for circumcision, thereby eliminating the possibility of injury during assembly or disassembly of the scalpel handle and blade. The sharps disposal container should be at arm's reach from the circumcision table. Using a scalpel blade without the handle should be avoided.

Syringes, Intravenous Catheters, and Lancets

Because hollow-bore needlesticks carry such a high risk and because such procedures are so common in obstetrics, the following section (also found in chapter 4) is reiterated here for emphasis.

Safety Syringes, Phlebotomy Devices, and Lancets

Hollow-bore needlesticks associated with venous access procedures and injuries from lancets may be significantly reduced by choosing appropriate equipment. A variety of intravenous catheters, phlebotomy devices, and lancets are available with features that can protect care givers by shielding or retracting the needle or lancet after use.

Needleless Intravenous Connection Systems

Obstetrical and surgical patients commonly require solutions and medications "piggybacked" into primary IV lines. Blood, seen or unseen, may back up into IV lines, making punctures by needles removed from IV connections a potential source of occupational transmission of bloodborne pathogens. Needleless IV connection systems with valves or plug-in or twist locking mechanisms may significantly reduce the hazard of needlesticks for surgical, obstetrical, and anesthesia personnel.

Blood Collection Tubes

Injecting blood through collection tube stoppers using an exposed needle should be avoided. Instead, shielded vacuum tubes or shielded phlebotomy syringes may be used. Plastic blood collection tubes and capillary tubes are preferable to glass to avoid breakage and the creation of sharp edges, which may cause injuries.

Disposal of Blood, Body Fluids and Tissue

Disposal of large volumes of blood, body fluids and tissue (i.e., suction canister contents and placentas) may be managed most efficiently using engineering controls such as encapsulation/solidification agents. The alternative, which is direct disposal by personnel who must be fully dressed with effective protective equipment, does not eliminate the risk of exposure through spills, splashes or aerosols.

Gloving for Venous Access Procedures

Gloves are appropriate for procedures involving the use of needles, IV catheters, or other sharp devices.

References/Suggested Readings

Rudnick J, Chamberland M, Panlilio A, et al. Blood contacts during obstetrical procedures. *Infect Control Hosp Epidemiol* 1994;15:349.

Notes

Hazards identified: _____

_____

_____

_____

_____

_____

_____

Planned changes: _____

_____

_____

_____

_____

_____

Current protocol for collection of cord blood and cord blood gases: _____

_____

_____

Current placement of personal protective equipment in the labor and delivery and operating room: _____

_____

_____

Current protocol for sharps disposal with vaginal delivery: _____

_____

_____

CHAPTER 13

Minimally Invasive Surgery

Old and New Hazards, Evolving Technology

From the standpoint of occupational exposure prevention, there are several potential benefits we may realize as a result of the growing shift from traditional to minimally invasive surgery. One is a general decrease in the number of sharps found on the sterile field. Another is cutting and other hazardous tasks occur mostly inside the patient, away from the fingers of surgical team members. Some old hazards, however, still remain and new ones have been introduced.

The three devices most responsible for sharps injuries in laparoscopic/endoscopic procedures are still suture needles, scalpel blades, and syringe needles. Blood aerosols created within the abdomen by laser and cautery present a new additional hazard. The American National Standard Institute (ANSI) found that electrosurgical devices and lasers produce the same types of airborne contamination, and recommended evacuation of smoke from all surgical sites. Intracardiac and intravascular balloon dilatation procedures have reduced the need for more invasive cardiothoracic and vascular procedures. Endometrial ablation procedures may totally avoid the invasive procedure of hysterectomy, but lasers and related technology have their own set of risks. It is possible that potentially safer technology, such as uterine balloon thermal ablation, may prove useful in this regard. The use of electrosurgical devices which seal vessels or tissue without the need for suturing may further reduce the incidence of needlesticks.

Safer Laparoscopic Access for Patients and Personnel

Injuries to the hands of personnel is possible during passing or handling of sharp trocars. Trocar injuries to patients are infrequent but often catastrophic, with injury to the major blood vessels or viscera. For this reason, many surgical subspecialists use either open technique or a variety of blunt trocars for initial abdominal access. Many gynecologic surgeons continue to use a blind approach to initial abdominal access, using a variety of sharp cutting trocars (some recessed or shielded), or conical blunt trocars. Cutting trocars which are shielded may be safer than those with exposed cutting surfaces. At the time of publication, blunt conical rounded disposable trocars which allow visualization, through a laparoscope, of each layer of the abdominal wall during entry had been recently introduced. Such devices, if proven effective and cost-effective, may provide an additional way to further reduce the risk of injury to patients and personnel.

Personal Protective Equipment

Although some surgical procedures may begin as minimally invasive, the potential for having to perform an open procedure exists; informed consent makes this clear to the patient. The O.R. team should also prepare accordingly and choose appropriate full protective barriers for *all* invasive procedures.

Use the following checklist to maximize exposure prevention during minimally invasive procedures:

Minimally Invasive Surgery Safety Checklist

❑ Pass trocars, needles, and other short sharps through a Neutral Zone.

❑ Pass long laparoscopic instruments that don't fit in the NZ, such as needle-tip cautery and sharp-pointed scissors, handle first and tip down.

❑ Place long-pointed cautery needles, hollow-bore needles or other long sharps into sleeve ports, on request, using two hands—preferably one person's hands—and then angle the handle toward the surgeon's waiting hand.

❑ Use shielded rather than exposed trocars and shielded needle systems wherever possible; blunt trocars may afford additional further protection.

❑ Blunt-tipped suture needles may be used effectively during laparoscopic hysterectomy and are considered a safer option for patient and surgeon (personal communication, Harry Reich, M.D.).

❑ Avoid sprayback; use trocar valves to protect anesthesia personnel as well as the surgical team.

❑ Periodically suction cautery smoke and laser plume to protect the patient from toxic gases.

❑ Aspirate all gas, fluid, and blood from the abdomen prior to closing.

Add to the list as you deem necessary.

References/Suggested Readings

American National Standard for the Safe Use of Lasers in Health Care Facilities, publication Z136.3. New York: ANSI 1988.

Jagger J, Beyea SC, Nicoll LH. AORN/BD/UVA multi-site clinical research study: Monitoring sharp object injuries blood and body fluid exposures in the O.R. Presentation at AORN Congress 4/10/97.

Notes

Hazards identified: _____

_____

_____

_____

_____

_____

_____

Planned changes: _____

_____

_____

_____

_____

_____

_____

Use of Neutral Zone: _____

_____

_____

Current protocol for passing long instruments: _____

_____

_____

Current protocol for aspiration of smoke and plume: _____

_____

_____

CHAPTER 14

Patients with Known Bloodborne Pathogens

All surgical patients must be treated as if they are infectious, and every patient deserves the same standard of care. Each healthcare worker deserves and should demand the same level of protection when performing his or her duties, regardless of the patient's known infectious state. If the integrated strategies outlined in the previous chapters are routinely and consistently applied, few additional measures will be required in cases where the patient is a known carrier of one or more bloodborne pathogens. The use of sharps will have already been markedly limited, and any sharps used will be managed as safely as possible. An additional advantage gained by having adopted a safer routine with *all* patients is that all members of the surgical team will have become familiar with the safer devices and techniques, and the added stress and danger of using unfamiliar equipment in a known dangerous situation is thereby avoided. Following the checklist below, therefore, is advisable whether the patient's infectious status is unknown or known:

❑ Develop an exposure prevention plan pre-operatively.

❑ Limit access to the room to necessary personnel. Crowding exacerbates the risk of exposures.

❑ Discuss any possible or planned deviations from usual techniques or protocols with the surgical team.

❑ Develop a written protocol and upgrade it with new technology and techniques.

❑ Strive to use *minimal* sharps during the procedure if feasible. This can often be done and obviate the need for cumbersome personal protective equipment.

❏ Utilize the principles of safe sharps management outlined in chapters 6, 7, 8, and 9. If scalpels are required, use only disposables.

❏ Use a smoke evacuator with electrocautery as well as laser.

❏ Use the most effective eye and face protection you can comfortably work with.

❏ Consider covering the neck area for additional protection. This is important for men who shave daily. Some male surgeons do not shave on surgery day to prevent skin breaks.

❏ Focus on safety with every hand motion and think before acting or speaking when sharps are in use.

Additional precautions may be useful, at the discretion of surgical team members, when the patient is known to harbor hepatitis C, HIV, or other bloodborne pathogens. Some are listed below; add to the list as necessary.

❏ Alert all members of the O.R. team.

❏ Discuss any possible or planned deviations from usual techniques or protocols with the surgical team.

❏ Strive to use *no* sharps during the procedure if feasible. This can often be done, obviating the need for cumbersome personal protective equipment.

❏ If any sharps are to be used, use the principles of safe sharps management outlined in chapters 6, 7, 8, and 9. If scalpels are required, use only disposables.

❏ Consider adding a third layer of gloves, with the outer layer elbow length.

❏ Change outer layer of gloves every hour to ensure barrier integrity.

❏ Consider using an electronic alarm system to indicate glove or gown breaches.

Routine Preoperative Testing

Routine preoperative serologic testing of surgical patients for HIV has not been recommended by the Public Health Service, nor by any medical or nursing organizations, for the following reasons:

1. Preoperative testing is considered a waste of resources and potentially dangerously misleading, as patients with early HIV infection will not test positive in the early window of seronegativity. Such patients have very high viral loads, similar to end stage AIDS patients, and their blood is highly infectious. Negative preoperative test results here could lead to a false sense of security. (However, as previously noted in chapter 4, post-exposure follow-up is greatly facilitated if *all surgical patients have, along with routine preoperative lab tests, a tube of blood drawn pre-operatively* to be held for possible HIV testing should an exposure occur. *A signed consent for HIV testing, also obtained pre-operatively, is another valid precaution.*)

2. Emergency patients have a greater chance of having HIV than elective surgery patients. Patients requiring emergency surgery may not be able to give consent for HIV testing. Additionally, the time required for testing of patients who need emergency surgery might delay their care.

3. The incidence of injuries and exposures to operating room personnel has been shown *not* to decrease despite personnel being aware that the patient has HIV or other serious disease. Factors that *do* lower the risk of exposure are the choices of equipment and the manner in which sharps are managed.

4. Many patients with chronic hepatitis C are undiagnosed, representing equal, if not more dangerous sources of exposure than HIV.

For the reasons stated, the use of a hierarchy of controls (the universal application of safer work practices and safer devices) is more beneficial than universal testing. *All* surgical patients, whether elective or emergency, must be treated as if they are infected and infectious.

References/Suggested Readings

Gerberding JL, Littell C, Tarkington A, Brown A, Schecter WP. Risk of exposure of surgical personnel to patients' blood during surgery at San Francisco General Hospital. *NEJM* 1990;322:1788–1793.

Notes

Hazards identified: _____

_____

_____

_____

_____

_____

_____

_____

Planned changes: _____

_____

_____

_____

Safety protocols in effect for all patients: _____

_____

_____

_____

Additional precautions for known infected patients: _____

_____

_____

_____

_____

_____

_____

_____

Administrative Support and Interaction

CHAPTER 15

The O.R. Management Team

Navigating the Winds of Change

Caught up as we are today in a time of rapid and relentless change, healthcare managers and workers have had no choice but to participate. The time of a reactive approach to adverse events in healthcare is gone; we have become proactive. Patient and worker safety, cost, and efficiency must now be addressed simultaneously. This is clearly a challenge of significant proportions that fortunately may be answered by using tools already in place.

By applying the tools of outcome management, quality assurance, and continuous quality improvement to exposure prevention as we do to patient care, we may gain control of this thorny problem. We must use these proven effective tools to monitor adverse events and outcomes in a collaborative work environment. The solution is at hand: We have the tools to communicate and educate, and we have access to safer technology.

Developing an Action Plan

Develop an action plan to prevent exposures and manage the environment. Take initiative and share ownership of appropriate decision making. Include a mission statement such as, "To provide a safe, functional, and effective surgical environment for patients and staff." Discuss the following areas:

- Individual responsibility

- Joint accountability
- Initiative
- Innovation
- Brainstorming
- Respect for diverse safe approaches
- Collaboration
- Continual improvement

Dealing With Denial

All members of the surgical team must come to understand and accept the simple truth that today, as with healthcare in general, the solution to exposure prevention is to do some things differently. We can control our own destiny but only by changing with the times. Driven by the evolution of occupational risk factors associated with bloodborne pathogens, everyone involved should consider themselves members of a task force working on exposure prevention.

Anyone who is not part of the solution must know they are part of the problem. As more operating room professionals adopt safer techniques and safer technology, the position of the minority who do not becomes more difficult to justify or defend. Negative factors such as habit and denial leading to dangerous behavior patterns will yield in the face of persistent communication, education, and safer technology.

Ensuring Adequate Protection for All

As noted in chapter 4, the range of personal protective equipment purchased by an institution should take into account the special needs of individuals. Personnel should be encouraged to voice those needs and to assume a share of the responsibility for their own protection. When a specific item does not meet the needs of a worker and training in correct application of the device does not solve the problem, additional or alternative equipment should be purchased.

Resources for Training and Education

Safety in the operating room demands daily attention and periodic maintenance. In the classroom, at in-services and elsewhere, many opportunities for exposure prevention exist. Educate staff in safe and effective protocols. Develop and publish standards to measure performance in managing and improving the environment. The following varied resources may be used effectively:

❏ In-services on new safety devices and updated safety protocols

❏ Workshops

❏ Small group discussions

❏ Periodic communication and updates on bloodborne pathogen risk and safety reminders:

  –Posters (see figure 15.1)

  –Memos

  –Flyers

  –Videotapes

❏ Education for all team members and newly added staff

❏ Mentoring of new personnel by experienced staff

❏ Encouragement of personnel to focus on exposure prevention throughout every procedure

❏ Communication among team members

❏ Provision of easy access to support and advice

❏ An appropriately tailored Safety Checklist posted in each room (see Appendix A)

Remind personnel great benefit may be derived from observing and documenting near-exposures as well as exposures. The "near-misses" are priceless learning opportunities and should be discussed at department meetings and in-services. This encourages brainstorming, an important component of continuous quality improvement (CQI).

The Role of Continuous Quality Improvement (Performance Improvement)

Either the hospital-wide or surgical CQI committee may facilitate the following functions:

❏ Trending of injury and exposure rates

❏ Facilitating reporting of exposures 24 hours a day

❑ Coordination of safety training and education

❑ Ensuring access to user-friendly technology for all

❑ Monitoring of compliance with safety protocols

The component steps of CQI are:

❑ Defining the problem at your hospital

❑ Gathering data on exposures

❑ Brainstorming solutions

❑ Identifying and evaluating strategic corrective interventions

❑ Communicating those interventions to the staff

❑ Training the staff on their correct application

❑ Seeking a volunteer or assigning a "safety champion" as a project coordinator and facilitator

❑ Measuring the effect on injury and exposure rates

❑ Measuring cost-effectiveness

❑ Documenting the daily universal use of personal protective equipment and safety protocols by personnel

❑ Identifying individuals with recurrent problems for special education, training, and discipline, if necessary

A summary game plan for creating a safer surgical environment using CQI is listed below:

1. Define the problem in your O.R. by documenting exposures.

2. Brainstorm and evaluate strategic interventions.

3. Train all staff in proper use of chosen strategies.

4. Measure effectiveness in reducing injuries and exposures.

5. Monitor the daily use of personal protective equipment, safety devices, and safety protocols by personnel.

6. Know how to access the safety marketplace.

BIOHAZARD   BIOHAZARD   BIOHAZARD

Blood and Body Fluids Safety Reminders
- Wear your PPE (and please remind teammates)
- Bloodborne pathogens are on the increase
- All blood is potentially infectious
- Standard Precautions for all patients
- Don't be part of the problem
- Be part of the solution
- Spread the word

When Using Sharps
- Focus
- Slow down
- Communicate
- Transfer safely
- Use instruments, not fingers
- Act as a team to prevent exposures
- Choose blunt alternatives when possible

Figure 15.1 O.R. poster

Copyrighted material. This page may be copied, showing the information in this box. *Advanced Precautions for Today's O.R.*, Sweinbinder Publications LLC, PO Box 11988, Atlanta, GA 30355. Updated versions and additional resources available.

Notes

Resources for training and education: _____

_____

_____

_____

_____

_____

_____

Add to the checklist in this chapter as necessary _____

_____

_____

_____

_____

_____

_____

Involvement of CQI team _____

_____

_____

_____

_____

_____

_____

CHAPTER 16

The Risk Management Team

Exposure prevention is essentially and intrinsically a risk-management issue. Every injury and bloodborne exposure is a potential liability, and most are preventable. Moreover, a large percentage of scalpel and suture needle injuries in surgery are inflicted by one healthcare worker on another. Additionally, although infrequent, transmission of bloodborne pathogens from healthcare worker to patient has been well documented. Such an occurrence could be a potential public relations nightmare for any institution. Although personal safety and protection is on the minds of all healthcare workers in this era of evolving deadly bloodborne pathogens, the necessary focus on safety can be lost in the moment of caring for surgical patients, especially in emergent situations. Adopting a comprehensive and detailed injury and exposure prevention plan for the operating room and delivery room simultaneously provides an effective risk-management plan as well.

Facilitating OSHA Compliance in the O.R.

Risk management and compliance with OSHA requirements also go hand-in-hand. The dual purpose of this book is to raise the level of exposure prevention and facilitate compliance with OSHA regulations in the operating room, a uniquely hazardous work site. Universal Precautions, Standard Precautions, and the recommendations in OSHA's Bloodborne Pathogen Standard and Final Rule are all *insufficiently specific* to address the special hazards found in the O.R. A detailed, integrated strategy for preventing sharps injuries and resulting bloodborne exposures, such as the one described in this book, is helpful.

For optimal success, positive change must occur at three levels: the individual, the surgical team, and the institution. The methodology of this book is, first, to make all members of the surgical team fully aware of the bloodborne pathogen hazard inherent in every invasive procedure and of currently available technology and techniques for injury and exposure prevention. Once individuals have chosen from the list of safe options on a personal level, the second level of prevention must be realized at the team level. This requires constant focus, good verbal communication, and teamwork.

The third tier of exposure prevention must come at the institutional level. *Herein lies the opportunity to oversee lasting change*, and fortunately the tools necessary to accomplish this are already in place. Those tools include detailed documentation and trending of site-specific exposures and near-exposures, periodic training and education, monitoring of compliance with established protocols, comprehensive product evaluation, and perhaps most powerful of all, continuous quality improvement.

The various hospital committees that address these issues must ultimately come together, with their gathered information and expertise under the umbrella and direction of CQI. The risk manager—rightfully one of the innate driving forces behind the project—is clearly a key participant in the continuous quality improvement process. Personnel from infection control, occupational health, O.R. management, product evaluation, and purchasing are essential spokes in the wheel. It is also critically important for O.R. professionals—the *users* of dangerous devices in hazardous situations—to actively participate in the evaluation of safer technology and techniques, and to serve on the appropriate committees. Surgeons, in particular, are busy people who often have good excuses for missing meetings; regardless, they must be relentlessly sought out for their input.

Whereas budgets are increasingly being slashed in many areas of hospital management, today more than ever, efficient expenditures for injury and exposure prevention must remain an institutional risk-management priority. Resources must be directed where they do the most good. For instance, if routine serologic testing of surgical patients (and O.R. professionals) for HIV and hepatitis C should become mandated in the future, substantial resources will have been wasted with no impact on injury and exposure rates. Expensive practices such as universal testing will only raise healthcare overhead, doing little to solve the problem; rather, resources should be directed toward *specific, effective prevention measures*.

Unreported Injuries and Exposures

Although the focus of this book is prevention, exposures cannot be totally eliminated. If despite our best efforts an exposure occurs, it should be reported; non-reporting could have disastrous consequences. In the case of significant exposure to HIV, initiation of post-exposure prophylaxis should begin within one to two hours, according to the U.S. Public Health Service (see Appendix B). Timely and accurate data collection following an exposure helps to ensure the exposed healthcare worker receives prompt and appropriate treatment and a clearly outlined course of follow-up.

Workers are more likely to report their injuries and exposures if a well-established and known plan is in place. Currently, computerized systems are being developed which may facilitate immediate and direct reporting by the exposed worker and facilitate appropriate counseling and follow-up.

Notes

Action plan for injury and exposure prevention: _____

_____

_____

_____

_____

_____

_____

_____

_____

_____

_____

CQI team: _____

_____

_____

_____

_____

_____

_____

_____

_____

_____

_____

_____

CHAPTER 17

The Product Evaluation and Purchasing Team

Today's changing healthcare environment is increasingly dominated by managed care and capitation. Institutions are challenged to simultaneously protect healthcare workers and patients from the increasing risk of exposure to bloodborne pathogens, cut costs, and locate needed medical devices and protective equipment in a rapidly changing industry. Reducing the incidence of exposures to bloodborne pathogens has become a significant economic incentive.

Safety Product Evaluation

Devices and systems designed to protect healthcare workers from injury and exposure to blood should undergo a thorough and effective evaluation. Acceptance by intended users is facilitated when they understand they are at risk for injury and when they have direct input into the selection process. O.R. professionals, the users of devices or systems intended for hazard reduction, should play a major role in their selection and deployment. An adequate supply of the device under evaluation is essential to avoid lack of interest among the users. Removing older similar devices, while keeping them available upon request, allows a more thorough evaluation of the new safety device and facilitates acceptance. The scheme for product evaluation proposed by Chiarello calls for a comprehensive and appropriate mix of team members. Surgeons, obstetricians, O.R. and O.B. managers, infection control and occupational health personnel, risk managers, materials managers, and administrative fiscal managers should be represented on the committee, and final purchasing decisions should not be made without the input of all.

In recent years, numerous products designed to reduce the risk of exposures have become commercially available. As "safety devices" are evaluated it will become apparent some work well and some do not. Critical evaluation will also reveal some might actually increase rather than decrease risk if improperly employed, thereby highlighting the importance of training all potential users before releasing devices for large-scale evaluation or general use.

Although some companies provide free samples, this is not always the case. A budget line item should exist for the testing and evaluation of new safety products.

Guidelines for product evaluation include:
- Define injury and exposure rates at your institution.
- Plan a trial in the appropriate clinical setting.
- Train users before trial.
- Limit evaluations to one device at a time.
- Allow sufficient time for users to try devices.
- Use a new device as a "default," with the old device available only by special request.
- Involve all potential users.
- Assess the results of the trial, including injury and exposure rates, user satisfaction, and critical comments.
- Monitor patient outcomes.

Questions to be answered during product evaluation:
- Were enough new devices available initially and throughout the trial to allow adequate evaluation by enough users?
- Was feedback obtained from all users?
- Was adequate training provided to instruct the users in the correct use of the device, particularly if incorrect use might introduce additional risk?
- Was a videotape or some other type of enduring resource provided to facilitate training and education of current and future personnel?

- If the device is complex, are there alternative devices available that are intrinsically safer, with fewer moving parts, or where activation of the safety feature is not required by the user?
- Are there characteristics of the device that would make the device dangerous in certain situations? If so, what do potential users need to know to compensate for this?
- Does cost-effectiveness analysis consider direct and indirect costs as well as savings?

Product performance should continue to be tracked following purchase to uncover any use problems or defects not discovered before purchase. Consultation with knowledgeable industry experts regarding future trends in the development of safety equipment may be useful.

The following are keys to making a purchasing decision:
- Use brainstorming.
- Utilize experts, consultants, and vendors as resources.
- Use a multidisciplinary team.
- Reward the team (bonuses, awards, etc.) for positive action.

Decisions on whether to purchase new devices should be based on the following factors:
- The effectiveness of the proposed product in reducing risk
- The cost and effectiveness of currently used technology
- The cost of replacement of existing technology
- The projected cost savings generated by preventing future injuries and exposures

It cannot be emphasized enough that final purchasing decisions should not be made without the input of all departments. Ensuring access to user-friendly and safe technology for all of the workers at the institution is essential. Meeting this goal sometimes requires expanding the institution's selection of personal protective equipment and other safety engineered devices.

Effectiveness and Cost-Effectiveness

While the cost of new equipment is relatively easy to capture, the savings from appropriate and effective usage may be more difficult to define. Because bloodborne exposures are very costly events, a logical assumption is that devices most effective in lowering exposure rates are likely to be the most cost-effective. Although there will be exceptions to this, it is a good principle to bear in mind. As the insurance industry applies pressure on healthcare systems to provide more services for less reimbursement, the expanded use of protective equipment and safety devices may be appropriately viewed by institutions as an investment in the protection of their employees and the patients they serve.

Accessing the "Safety" Marketplace

The large number of suppliers of safety equipment and continual change within the industry are factors that present challenges to hospital purchasing services in search of specific equipment or services. As with medical supplies in general, there is no single source. Rapidly increasing numbers of companies sell or distribute personal protective equipment and safety-engineered surgical devices and provide consulting or educational services. New companies enter the market every year—some with only one or two products to offer—yet some of those products may fill a significant need. Companies regularly leave the marketplace as well, and specific products may be acquired by one company from another, further adding to confusion about purchasing specific devices.

To facilitate access to the growing spectrum of safety devices and services, the current edition of a convenient listing of safety products, manufacturers, distributors, and providers of services should be consulted.

References/Suggested Readings

Laufer FN, Chiarello LA. Application of cost-effectiveness methodology to the consideration of needle stick prevention technology. *AJIC* 1994;22:75–82.

Chiarello LA. Practice forum: Selection of needlestick prevention devices: A conceptual framework for approaching product evaluation. *AJIC* 1995;23:6;386–395.

Notes

Hazards identified: _____

_____

_____

_____

_____

_____

_____

Products to be evaluated: _____

_____

_____

_____

_____

_____

_____

Projected cost savings: _____

_____

_____

_____

_____

_____

_____

CHAPTER 18

The Infection Control Team

Infection control professionals, along with epidemiologists, have been at the forefront of the exposure prevention movement since the beginning of recognition of the problem, and they will continue to be instrumental in gathering data on evolving bloodborne pathogens, injury and exposure patterns, and effectiveness of selected interventions. In a five-year study (Haiduven et al) of needlestick injuries from 1986 to 1990, additional needle disposal containers were added to patient care areas as close to the point of use as possible. The rates of reduction of needlesticks were communicated to personnel each year and extensive educational programs were conducted annually, resulting in a significant annual decrease in injuries. There was a 60% overall needlestick reduction rate over five years, including an 89% reduction of injuries from recapping. The authors used an effective three-pronged approach to significantly decrease needlestick injuries in healthcare workers: (1) more convenient placement of needle disposal containers, (2) periodic communication of findings to personnel, and (3) continuing education.

Although this landmark study was not conducted in a surgical setting, it is a useful model. If all we had to worry about in surgery was safe disposal of sharps, exposure prevention would be a relatively simpler matter. In the complex surgical environment, however, we clearly face a much broader challenge. The lesson learned from the Haiduven study is that providing convenient access to safer technology, periodic communication with those at risk, and continuing education will serve us well in our quest for a safer workplace.

Occupational Health Resources

At each hospital, occupational health professionals have the responsibility—and indeed the fortuitous opportunity—to gather valuable data on site-specific and worker-specific injuries and exposures. Although these data must remain confidential, they serve the vital purpose of identifying existing and evolving exposure patterns at a given institution. These data become the basis for identifying problems, thus enabling the selection of effective interventions to reduce exposures.

The Infection Control Committee

To effectively address the problem of exposure prevention, membership of the infection control committee should include representatives from surgery, obstetrics, O.R. and O.B. management, risk management, and administration. Data on exposures can be provided to the CQI committee for shared interaction, brainstorming, and problem resolution.

More and more hospitals and centers are now sharing their information on occupational exposures with national and international data banks, such as EPINet, and the newly introduced EPINet O.R. Analyzed pooled data from these resources is providing important information on incidence rates and patterns of exposures that may subsequently be used by all institutions to lower individual exposure rates.

Sharing Data With Those at Risk

Front-line healthcare workers—the people at risk at every institution—must know there is an ongoing problem that must be addressed on a daily basis. If, for example, there are 50 O.R. professionals at an institution and there was only one (self-inflicted) exposure this month, 49 individuals probably have no knowledge of the incident. Without compromising confidentiality, it helps if all 50 workers are periodically reminded of this ongoing problem.

The processes of *continuing education and periodic communication* lead to an appropriate level of awareness, and to rejection of inappropriate denial. With a continuing hazard in the workplace, everyone should understand individual and team effort is required and managerial and administrative help is available.

References/Suggested Readings

Haiduven DJ, DeMaio TM, Stevens DA. A five-year study of needlestick injuries: significant reduction associated with communication, education, and convenient placement of sharps containers. *Infect Control Hosp Epidemiol* 1992;13:265–271.

Advances in Exposure Prevention. Published by the International Healthcare Worker Safety Research and Resource Center at the University of Virginia. For subscriber information, call customer service: (804) 924-5159. Web site: http://www.med.virginia.edu/~epinet

Notes

Injury and exposure trends identified: _____

_____

_____

_____

_____

_____

_____

Action plan: _____

_____

_____

_____

_____

_____

_____

CQI team: _____

_____

_____

_____

_____

_____

_____

_____

Safety Checklists for the Operating Room and Delivery Room

Purpose and Function of Safety Checklists

Before every commercial airplane takeoff and landing, the flight crew goes through a checklist to ensure all safety devices are activated and established safety protocols are being followed. We have found it helpful to adopt this practice in our surgical, obstetrical, and other invasive medical settings.

You will doubtless find the type of procedure being performed and the personnel involved will dictate the composition of your checklist. Some form of basic checklist is applicable for all types of surgery, but additional items or modifications, appropriate to particular procedures or work sites, may be added. The checklist for cataract extraction, for example, will be shorter than the checklists for hip replacement, cesarean section, liver transplantation, or cardiopulmonary bypass as these procedures have increased numbers of personnel and use additional hazardous devices.

The following checklists are suggested as models. Please copy and modify to meet your specific needs. They should be continuously updated and revised as new technology emerges and new techniques are devised. Posting the list on or near the door of each operating and delivery room will serve as an important daily reminder, allowing safer behavior patterns to become second nature.

Operating Room Safety Checklist
Post at scrub sinks or OR doors.

1. **Personal protective equipment:**
   - ❏ Head wear with appropriate coverage
   - ❏ Eye and face protection in place
   - ❏ Neck protection as indicated
   - ❏ Appropriate gown
   - ❏ Impervious boots/shoe covers
   - ❏ Double gloves/special gloves/glove liners as indicated
   - ❏ Waterproof drapes/pouches as indicated

2. **Work practice controls:**
   - ❏ Neutral Zone selected and deployed
   - ❏ Surgeon (   ) right-handed (   ) left-handed
   - ❏ Assistant (   ) right-handed (   ) left-handed
   - ❏ Appropriate suture needle selection (blunt if applicable)
   - ❏ Appropriate retractor selection (blunt if applicable)
   - ❏ Suture assist devices
   - ❏ Disposable scalpels if appropriate
   - ❏ Smoke evacuation equipment available and functioning

3. **Sharps management and disposal devices available:**
   - ❏ Needle parking devices
   - ❏ Needle capping devices
   - ❏ Scalpel blade manipulators
   - ❏ Sharps disposal/counting boxes

Delivery Room Safety Checklist
Post at scrub sinks or OR doors.

1. **Personal protective equipment:**
   - ❏ Head wear with appropriate coverage
   - ❏ Eye and face protection in place
   - ❏ Neck protection as indicated
   - ❏ Appropriate gown
   - ❏ Impervious boots/shoe covers
   - ❏ Double gloves/extended cuff gloves/glove liners as indicated
   - ❏ Waterproof drapes/pouches as indicated

2. **Work practice controls:**
   - ❏ Appropriate suture needle selection (blunt if applicable)
   - ❏ Appropriate retractor selection (blunt if applicable)
   - ❏ Suture assist devices

3. **Sharps management and disposal devices available:**
   - ❏ Needle parking (suture assist) devices (if using sharp needles)
   - ❏ Needle capping devices
   - ❏ Sharps disposal/counting box

APPENDIX B

Summary of Public Health Service Recommendations for Management of Occupational Exposure to Blood and Body Fluids

Healthcare professionals who work in exposure-prone areas, especially operating room professionals, should know how to respond immediately to an exposure incident and know what their options are. Although preventing blood exposures is the primary means of preventing occupationally acquired human immunodeficiency virus (HIV) infection and hepatitis C virus (HCV) infection, appropriate post-exposure management measures, including HIV Post-exposure Prophylaxis (PEP), are important elements of workplace safety. On May 15, 1998 the Centers for Disease Control and Prevention (CDC) published updated guidelines and recommendations to assist clinicians caring for occupationally exposed health-care workers (HCWs) (see reference at end of Appendix B). Much of the information in Appendix B is from those guidelines and recommendations, reproduced here to help HCWs at risk of exposure to understand the process of post-exposure management in its present form. Further updates from the CDC will follow as more information becomes available on the efficacy and toxicity of antiretroviral drugs used for HIV PEP.

Administrative Considerations
Experienced clinically trained medical or nursing personnel should assess the severity of an exposure. The initiation of a basic PEP regimen

necessitates knowledge or experience in clinical epidemiology, infection control, occupational health, or the clinical treatment of HIV. Decisions about HIV PEP are particularly complex if protease inhibitors (PIs) are used or there is concern about drug-resistant virus. Thus, the CDC strongly encourages expert consultation when prescribing PEP, and PEP protocols should list the names of readily available resources for consultation and could include policies that require infectious disease evaluation before prescribing an expanded antiretroviral regimen. However, these efforts should not delay initial implementation of PEP where it is appropriate.

Recommendations for the Management of Potentially Exposed HCWs

The following steps should be carried out immediately after an exposure or as soon as it is recognized an exposure has occurred:

1. Treat the exposure site.
2. Report the exposure.
3. Assessment of the risk of bloodborne pathogen infection by appropriate clinical personnel.

The policies at individual hospitals and institutions, guided by their infection control and occupational health departments, may include additions to the most current Public Health Service guidelines and recommendations.

Treatment of the Exposure Site

- *Percutaneous/Skin:* Wash puncture wounds, cuts or exposed intact or non-intact skin with soap and running water. There is no evidence that using antiseptics for wound care or expressing blood from a sharps injury wound further reduce the risk of HIV infection; however, the use of antiseptics is not contraindicated. The application of caustic agents such as bleach is not recommended.
- *Mucous membrane:* Flush oral and nasal mucosa with water. Irrigate eyes with clean water, saline, or appropriate sterile solution.
- *Reporting:* Report the exposure to the occupational health department or the appropriate department manager or supervisor

according to facility protocol. If indicated, PEP should be initiated promptly, within one or two hours post-exposure.

Assessment of infection risk and appropriate counseling should be promptly initiated to determine the need for HIV PEP and additional follow-up.

Assessment of Infection Risk

After an occupational exposure, the source-person and the exposed HCW should be evaluated to determine the need for HIV PEP. Rapid HIV tests can assist healthcare providers who must make immediate decisions about initiating HIV prophylaxis in healthcare workers after occupational exposure. A study by the CDC indicated substantially improved delivery of counseling and testing when a rapid test for HIV screening was used. A commercially available rapid test to detect HIV antibody (Single Use Diagnostic System HIV-1 Test, Murex Corp, Norcross, GA) can be performed in an average of ten minutes. The sensitivity and specificity of rapid assays are comparable to those of enzyme immunoassays (EIAs), which take approximately 1 to 2 weeks. A negative rapid test does not require further testing. A reactive test must be confirmed by a supplemental test. Follow-up for hepatitis B virus and hepatitis C virus infections also should be conducted in accordance with CDC recommendations (see *Additional Follow-Up* below).

Evaluation of exposure. The exposure is evaluated for potential to transmit HIV based on the type of body substance involved and the route and severity of the exposure.

Evaluation and testing of an exposure source. The source patient whose blood or body fluids are the source of an exposure is evaluated for HIV infection, severity of infection (viral load), or risk factors for infection by appropriate testing. If complete information is not immediately available, initiation of PEP, if indicated, should not be delayed. Changes in the PEP regimen can be made after PEP has been started, as appropriate. Testing of the source material or patient should be as prompt as the law will allow.

Determining the need for HIV PEP is done by the clinician caring for the exposed worker in three steps:

Step 1. **Determine the EXPOSURE CODE** (EC) by categorizing the source material and type of exposure. The EC scale of risk ranges from 1 to 3 in severity and is based on the following factors:

- Blood, body fluid, or other potentially infectious material (OPIM) exposure to mucous membrane or skin, integrity compromised, *or* to intact skin only, *or* percutaneous exposure.
- Volume and duration of exposure: less severe (solid needle/superficial scratch) *or* more severe (e.g., large-bore needle, deep puncture, visible blood on device, or needle used in source patient's artery or vein).

Step 2. **Determine the HIV STATUS CODE** (HIV SC) by categorizing the HIV status of the exposure source. The HIV SC scale of risk is: 1, 2, or unknown. It is based on the following factors:

- Exposure source HIV negative *or* HIV positive *or* status unknown *or* source unknown.
- Lower titer exposure (e.g., asymptomatic and high CD4 count) *or* higher titer exposure (e.g., advanced AIDS, primary HIV infection, high or increasing viral load, or low CD4 count).

Step 3. **Determine the PEP recommendation** using Steps 1 and 2 to arrive at one of the following recommendations:

PEP may not be warranted. Exposure type does not pose a known risk for HIV transmission. Whether or not the risk for drug toxicity outweighs the benefit of PEP should be decided by the exposed healthcare worker and his or her treating clinician.

Consider basic regimen. Exposure type poses a negligible risk for HIV transmission. A high HIV titer in the source may justify consideration of PEP. Whether or not the risk for drug toxicity outweighs the benefit of PEP should be decided by the exposed healthcare worker and treating clinician.

Recommend basic regimen. Most HIV exposures are in this category; no increased risk for HIV transmission has been observed but use of PEP is appropriate.

Recommend expanded regimen. Exposure type represents an increased HIV transmission risk.

Clinical Evaluation and Baseline Testing of Exposed Healthcare Workers

Clinical evaluation and baseline testing of exposed healthcare workers for HIV is performed if the source is HIV positive. If the source person is seronegative for HIV, baseline testing or further follow-up is not necessary, unless the source patient has recently engaged in behaviors associated with a risk for HIV transmission. In those cases, baseline and follow-up HIV-antibody testing at three and/or six months postexposure should be considered. Exposed workers in this category are advised to take appropriate precautions, including safe sex, avoidance of pregnancy or breast feeding, and so forth until completion of the surveillance period. Psychological counseling should be offered to exposed workers and family members as needed.

HIV PEP

The following recommendations apply to situations where an HCW has had an exposure to a source person with HIV or where information suggests there is a likelihood the source person is HIV infected. These recommendations are based on the risk for HIV infection after different types of exposure and limited data regarding efficacy and toxicity of PEP. Because most occupational HIV exposures do not result in transmission of HIV, potential toxicity must be carefully considered when prescribing PEP. When possible, these recommendations should be implemented in consultation with persons having expertise in antiretroviral therapy and HIV transmission.

Explaining PEP to HCWs

Recommendations for chemoprophylaxis should be explained to HCWs who have sustained occupational HIV exposures. In exposures for which PEP is considered appropriate, HCWs should be informed of the following:

1. Knowledge about the efficacy and toxicity of drugs used for PEP is limited.

2. Only ZDV has been shown to prevent HIV transmission in humans.

3. There is no data to address whether adding other antiretroviral drugs provides any additional benefit for PEP, but experts recom-

mend combination drug regimens because of increased potency and concerns about drug-resistant virus.

4. Data regarding toxicity of antiretroviral drugs in persons without HIV infection or in pregnant women is limited for ZDV and not known regarding other antiretroviral drugs.

5. Any or all drugs for PEP may be declined by the HCW. HCWs who have HIV occupational exposures for which PEP is not recommended should be informed that the potential side effects and toxicity of taking PEP outweigh the negligible risk of transmission posed by the exposure.

Factors in Selection of a PEP Regimen

Selection of the PEP regimen should consider the comparative risk represented by the exposure and information about the exposure source, including history of and response to antiretroviral therapy based on clinical response, CD4 + T-lymphocyte counts, viral load measurements, and current disease stage. Most HIV exposures will warrant only a two-drug regimen, usually ZDV and 3TC. The addition of a third drug, usually a protease inhibitor, should be considered for exposures that pose an increased risk of transmission or where resistance to the other drugs used for PEP is known or suspected.

Timing of PEP Initiation

PEP should be initiated as soon as possible. The interval within which PEP should be started for optimal efficacy is not known. Animal studies demonstrated the importance of starting PEP within hours after an exposure. To ensure timely access to PEP, an occupational exposure should be regarded as an urgent medical concern and PEP started as soon as possible after the exposure (i.e., within a few hours rather than days). If there is a question about which antiretroviral drugs to use or whether to use two or three drugs, it is probably better to start ZDV and 3TC immediately than to delay PEP administration. Although animal studies suggest that PEP probably is not effective when started later than 24 to 36 hours post-exposure, the interval after which there is no benefit from PEP for humans is undefined. Therefore, if appropriate for the exposure, PEP should be started even when the interval since exposure exceeds 36 hours. Initiating therapy after a longer interval (e.g., one to two weeks) may be considered for exposures that represent an increased risk for transmission. Even if infection is not prevented, early treatment of acute HIV infection may be beneficial. The optimal duration of PEP is unknown. Because four weeks of ZDV appeared protective in HCWs, PEP probably should be administered for four weeks, if tolerated.

PEP if Serostatus of Source Person is Unknown

If the source person's HIV serostatus is unknown at the time of exposure (including when the source is HIV negative but may have had a recent HIV exposure), use of PEP should be decided on a case-by-case basis, after considering the type of exposure and the clinical and/or epidemiologic likelihood of HIV infection in the source. If these considerations suggest a possibility for HIV transmission and HIV testing of the source is pending, it is reasonable to initiate a two-drug PEP regimen until laboratory results have been obtained and later modify or discontinue the regimen accordingly.

PEP if Exposure Source is Unknown

If the exposure source is unknown, use of PEP should be decided on a case-by-case basis. Consideration should include the severity of the exposure and the epidemiologic likelihood the HCW was exposed to HIV.

Follow-Up of HCWs Exposed to HIV
Post-exposure Testing

HCWs with occupational exposure to HIV should receive follow-up counseling, post-exposure testing, and medical evaluation regardless of whether they receive PEP. HIV-antibody testing should be performed for at least 6 months post-exposure (e.g., at 6 weeks, 12 weeks, and 6 months). It is unclear whether an extended follow-up period (e.g., 12 months) is indicated in certain circumstances. Although rare instances of delayed seroconversion have been reported, the CDC's position is the infrequency of this occurrence does not warrant adding to HCWs anxiety by routinely extending the duration of post-exposure follow-up. Circumstances for which extending the duration of follow-up have been suggested include the use of highly potent antiretroviral regimens (i.e., more than two drugs) because of theoretical concerns that HIV seroconversion could be delayed or there was simultaneous exposure to

HCV. Data are insufficient for making a general recommendation in these situations. However, this should not preclude a decision to extend follow-up in an individual situation based on the clinical judgment of the HCW's healthcare provider. HIV testing should be performed on any HCW who has an illness compatible with an acute retroviral syndrome, regardless of the interval since exposure. HIV-antibody testing using EIA should be used to monitor for seroconversion.

Monitoring and Management of PEP Toxicity

If PEP is used, drug-toxicity monitoring should be performed at baseline and again two weeks after starting PEP. Minimally these should include a complete blood count and renal and hepatic chemical function tests. Monitoring for evidence of hyperglycemia should be included for HCWs whose regimen included any PI; if the HCW is receiving IDV, monitoring for crystalluria, hematuria, hemolytic anemia, and hepatitis also should be included. If toxicity is noted, modification of the regimen should be considered after expert consultation; further diagnostic studies may be indicated.

HCWs who fail to complete the recommended regimen often do so because of the side effects they experience (e.g., nausea and diarrhea). These symptoms often can be managed without changing the regimen by prescribing antimotility and antiemetic agents or other medications that target the specific symptoms. In other situations, modifying the dose interval (i.e., administering a lower dose of drug more frequently throughout the day, as recommended by the manufacturer), may help promote adherence to the regimen.

Counseling and Education

Although HIV infection following an occupational exposure occurs infrequently, the emotional impact of the exposure often is substantial. In addition, HCWs are given seemingly conflicting information. Although HCWs are told there is a low risk for HIV transmission, a four- week regimen of PEP is recommended and they are asked to commit to behavioral measures (i.e., sexual abstinence or condom use) to prevent secondary transmission, all of which influence their lives for several weeks to months. Therefore, access to persons who are knowledgeable about occupational HIV transmission and who can deal with the many concerns an HIV exposure may raise for the HCW is an important element of post-exposure management.

There is no need to modify an HCW's patient-care responsibilities to prevent transmission to patients based solely on an HIV exposure. If HIV seroconversion is detected, the HCW should be evaluated according to published recommendations for HIV-infected HCWs. (Reference: CDC. Recommendations for preventing transmission of human immunodeficiency virus and hepatitis B virus to patients during exposure-prone invasive procedures. MMWR 1991;40(no.RR-8).

Exposed HCWs should be advised to seek medical evaluation for any acute illness that occurs during the follow-up period. Such an illness, particularly if characterized by fever, rash, myalgia, fatigue, malaise, or lymphadenopathy, may be indicative of acute HIV infection but also may be due to a drug reaction or another medical condition.

Exposed HCWs who choose to take PEP should be advised of the importance of completing the prescribed regimen. Information should be provided about potential drug interactions and the drugs that should not be taken with PEP, the side effects of the drugs that have been prescribed, measures to minimize these effects, and the methods of clinical monitoring for toxicity during the follow-up period. They should be advised that the evaluation of certain symptoms should not be delayed (e.g., back or abdominal pain, pain on urination or blood in the urine, or symptoms of hyperglycemia (i.e., increased thirst and/or frequent urination).

Recommendations for the Selection of Drugs for PEP

The selection of a drug regimen for HIV PEP must strive to balance the risk for infection against the potential toxicity of the agent(s) used. Because PEP is potentially toxic, its use is not justified for exposures that pose a negligible risk for transmission. Also, there is insufficient evidence to recommend a highly active regimen for all HIV exposures. Therefore, two regimens for PEP are provided: a "basic" two-drug regimen that should be appropriate for most HIV exposures and an "expanded" three-drug regimen that should be used for exposures that pose an increased risk for transmission or where resistance to one or more antiretroviral agents is known or suspected. When possible, the regimens should be implemented in consultation with persons having expertise in antiretroviral treatment and HIV transmission.

This appendix is not intended as a treatment guide but rather as an educational reference for healthcare workers at risk of exposure so they can understand the process of post-exposure management in its present form. Therefore, specific drug regimens, dosages, toxicity profiles, side effects, and drug interactions are not reproduced here. This information may be found in the reference cited at the end of this appendix. Healthcare workers should immediately consult the appropriate clinician at their facility for the most expert and up-to-date advice in the event of an exposure.

Additional Follow-up
- Draw initial laboratory studies on exposed worker, which may include:
  1. Hepatitis B surface antibody.
  2. Hepatitis C antibody.
- Post-exposure recommendations may include:
  1. Hepatitis B vaccine.
  2. Hepatitis B immune globulin (HBIG).
- Document exposures on appropriate reporting forms. Post-exposure and follow-up lab work, coordinated by Occupational Health Service (OHS):
  1. Hepatitis B, Hepatitis C and HIV screens in three months if source patient is negative.
  2. Hepatitis C screen in three months and six months if source patient is positive.
- Healthcare workers seen in the emergency department should follow up with OHS the next business day. Healthcare workers will be counseled on all post-exposure lab results.

With exposures from a known source patient:
- The source patient must be counseled by the attending physician regarding laboratory testing as required by law. Exposure lab tests on source patient include: (after consent obtained, if required)

1. HIV testing.
2. Hepatitis B surface antigen.
3. Hepatitis C antibody.

- If source patient refuses to consent to HIV testing, immediately notify OHS.

Hepatitis C Post-Exposure Guidelines

The CDC has recommended institutions consider implementing policies and procedures for follow-up of workers after percutaneous or mucosal exposure to HCV-positive blood. Such policies might include:

- Baseline testing of the source patient for anti-HCV antibody.
- Baseline and six month follow-up testing of exposed workers for anti-HCV and alanine aminotransferase activity.

All anti-HCV results should be confirmed by supplemental accurate anti-HCV testing.

Prevention of exposure is the only effective strategy for preventing infection with hepatitis C for the following reasons:

- There is no post-exposure drug prophylaxis for hepatitis C.
- Immune globulin is ineffective for hepatitis C.

The CDC recommends institutions provide healthcare workers with accurate and up-to-date information on the risk and prevention of all bloodborne pathogens, including hepatitis C.

Hepatitis B Vaccination and Follow-Up

All operating room professionals are at risk of contact with blood; therefore, all should receive the hepatitis B vaccination if they have not received it during their training. Employers must offer vaccination free of charge to employee healthcare workers by federal law. Serologic screening is not required prior to vaccination.

There are no known adverse effects to immunizing someone who is already immune because of previous vaccination or previous infection. Modern vaccines are well tolerated and safe. Pregnancy is not a contraindication. Mild soreness at the injection site, fever, headache, or fatigue have been reported, but no severe adverse acute or chronic effects have been documented.

Three doses of 1 ml of vaccine are given intramuscularly; initially, at one month, and six months, preferably in the deltoid muscle. Vaccine recipients over the age of 30, those with impaired immune response, and those who received the vaccine in the buttock rather than the deltoid muscle may not sufficiently respond with adequate antibody formation. The series of three doses of vaccine, when given as above, is effective in over 95% of otherwise healthy young adults. Post-vaccination testing should be performed to demonstrate sufficient antibody formation. Healthcare workers who develop anti-HBs concentrations of 10 milli-international units per milliliter (mIUs/ml.) or greater after a primary vaccination series are fully protected against clinical illness and chronic infection. Those who demonstrate anti-HBs concentrations of less than 10 milli-international units per milliliter should be offered one to three additional doses of vaccine, and post-vaccination testing should be repeated. Responders to vaccination, demonstrated by seroconversion, are thought to be protected against infection even if antibody levels have fallen to nondetectable levels at the time of an exposure. Ongoing longitudinal studies of long-term protection have thus far shown that almost 50% of immunized adults lose detectable anti-HBs, but remain protected from acute and chronic infections for up to 14 years. An increase in antibody production (anamnestic response) is triggered by exposure to the natural virus following an exposure. Based on these findings, the CDC does not recommend booster doses of vaccine for health care workers whose immune status is normal and who have responded to vaccination.

Resources for Consultation

Clinicians who seek consultation on HIV PEP for assistance in managing an occupational exposure should access local experts as much as possible. In addition, the National Clinicians' Post-Exposure Prophylaxis Hotline (PEP-Line) assists clinicians. Telephone toll-free (888) 448-4911.

PEPNet (see Additional Resources) is designed to provide access via the Internet for clinicians caring for exposed personnel to current information about post-exposure prophylaxis for preventing infection with HIV and other bloodborne viruses after exposure. Clinicians caring for exposed personnel should refer to manufacturers' full prescribing information for dosing and other information. PEPNet is maintained by the Epidemiology and Prevention Interventions Center (EPI Center) at the University of California, San Francisco (UCSF) and San Francisco General Hospital (SFGH). The treatment information provided by PEPNet is adapted from several sources including current PHS/ CDC guidelines for managing occupational exposures and guidelines for managing HIV-infected patients prepared by various consensus groups and is subject to change when new data become available.

References:

Center for Disease control and Prevention. Public Health Service Guidelines for the Management of Health-Care Worker Exposures to HIV and Recommendations for Post-exposure Prophylaxis. MMWR 1998;47(No. RR-7):Inclusive page numbers.

Centers for Disease Control and Prevention. Update: HIV counseling and testing using rapid tests—United States, 1995, *MMWR* 1998;47(11):211-214.

Please refer to the section *Additional Resources* for sources of updated information from the CDC.

Summary of OSHA Regulations Relevant to the Operating Room

OSHA Regulations

Congress enacted the Occupational Safety and Health Act and the Occupational Safety and Health Administration (OSHA) in 1970 to protect workers from unsafe and unhealthy conditions in the workplace. OSHA's regulations apply to employers and employees. OSHA has the authority to conduct unannounced workplace inspections and may assess civil or criminal penalties for failure to comply.

In 1991 OSHA issued regulations on occupational exposure to blood-borne pathogens designed to minimize the transmission of HIV, hepatitis, and other agents. The regulations cover all employees where workers could be reasonably anticipated to come into contact with blood and other potentially infectious materials on the job.

To comply with the regulations, healthcare employers are required to prepare a written Exposure Control Plan to eliminate or minimize employee exposure to blood-borne pathogens through blood, semen, vaginal secretions, peritoneal fluid, amniotic fluid, any bodily fluid visibly contaminated with blood, all body fluids in which it is impossible to differentiate between the body fluids, or any unfixed human tissue or organ (living or dead). The Exposure Control Plan requires employers to adopt the use of *Universal precautions, Engineering Controls, Work Practice Controls, and Personal Protective Equipment.*

OSHA Compliance Directive (CPL 2-2.44D)
November 5, 1999

Employers are required to update their written Exposure Control Plan to reflect significant improvements in technology in the growing market of safer medical devices between 1991 and 1999 and the effectiveness of these engineering controls. The Compliance Directive establishes policies and provides clarification to ensure uniform inspection procedures to enforce the Occupational Exposure to Bloodborne Pathogens Standard. This federal program change applies OSHA-wide; all states are expected to have standards, enforcement policies and procedures which are at least as effective.

Engineering Controls and Work Practices: The Compliance Directive clarifies the responsibility of employers to implement effective engineering controls to reduce sharps injuries. Effective engineering controls include the use of devices to prevent percutaneous injuries before, during, or after use through safer design features. Examples listed include blunt suture needles, needleless IV connectors and self-sheathing needles or syringes. Where engineering controls will reduce employee exposure either by removing, eliminating or isolating the hazard, they must be used. OSHA does not advocate the use of one particular device over another, but expects employers and users to use CDC studies of efficacy, pilot tests by the employer or data available in published studies to choose from available safer devices and implement them. Work practices referred to include no-hands passing of sharps. A detailed occupational exposure log must be kept and made available to OSHA inspectors.

Training and Education: Employers, including hospitals and physicians and/or their professional corporations, must train and educate employees (operating room staff and physicians) who use implemented engineering controls and work practices, to ensure acceptance and proper use by employees. If a combination of engineering controls and work practices used by the employer does not eliminate or minimize exposure, OSHA's instructions to its field inspectors are to cite the employer for failing to use engineering and work practice controls.

Liability of Surgeons/Physicians/Professional Corporations to Citation: In the section defining Multi-Employer and Related Worksites (pages

5-7 of the OSHA document CPL 2-2.44D), OSHA states that physicians and healthcare professionals who have established an independent practice may be employers or employees. Physicians who are unincorporated sole proprietors or partners in a bona fide partnership are employers for purposes of the Occupational Safety and Health Act, and may be cited if they employ at least one employee (such as a technician or secretary). Such physician-employers may be cited if they create or control bloodborne pathogens hazards that expose employees at hospitals or other sites where they have staff privileges. Physicians may be employed by a hospital or other healthcare facility or may be members of a professional corporation and conduct some of their activities at host employer sites (e.g.; hospitals, surgicenters, birthing centers) where they have staff privileges. Where professional corporations are the employers of their physician-members, professional corporations may be cited for exposure of its physicians and other workers at a host employer site.

Summary: Employers, including hospitals, physicians who provide surgical and obstetrical services at host facilities where they have staff privileges, and their professional corporations are required to update their existing exposure control plan, choose and implement effective engineering and work practices from the broadening market of safety devices, and effectively eliminate or minimize occupational exposures. To receive a hard copy of the 263 page document (DIRECTIVES NUMBER: CPL 2-2.44D), call the OSHA Office of Health Compliance Assistance (202) 693-2190. To download the document, visit the OSHA web site at www.osha.gov.

Federal Needlestick Safety and Prevention Act (S 3067)
October, 2000

The United States Congress passed the Needlestick Safety and Prevention Act (S 3067) on October 26, 2000, mandating that the 1991 OSHA Bloodborne Pathogens Standard (29 CFR1930.1030) be revised to require the use of safety-engineered sharp devices.

The law states that "modification of the bloodborne pathogens standard is appropriate to set forth in greater detail its requirement that employers identify, evaluate, and make use of effective safer medical devices." Its main provisions are:

(1) A revised and expanded definition of "engineering controls" in the bloodborne pathogens standard that includes "safer medical devices, such as sharps with engineered sharps injury protection and needleless systems."

(2) A definition of safety devices as "a non-needle sharp or a needle device with a built-in safety feature or mechanism that effectively reduces the risk of an exposure incident."

(3) A definition of "needleless systems as "a device that does not use needles for collection of bodily fluids or withdrawal of body fluids after initial venous or arterial access is established".

(4) A new requirement that exposure control plans include evaluation of safety devices. They must be updated as necessary to "reflect changes in technology that eliminate or reduce exposure to bloodborne pathogens" and "document consideration and implementation of appropriate commercially available and effective safer medical devices."

(5) A requirement that sharps injury logs be kept, in addition to the OSHA 200 log. The sharps injury log must include detailed information on the injury, including the "type and brand of device involved in the incident, the department or work area where the exposure incident occurred, and an explanation of how the incident occurred."

(6) A requirement that employers involve frontline health care workers when evaluating and selecting safer devices.

The bill includes a provision that the usual hearings process for amending an existing OSHA standard be bypassed, and the law will be in effect 90 days after the revised standard has been published in the Federal Register.

States with "state OSHA plans" (about half the states) are required to have regulations that are "at least as effective" as federal OSHA's, so these states will have to revise their bloodborne pathogens standard to reflect these new requirements.

To download a copy of the bill, go to www.senate.gov, scroll down to "Bill Search," type in S. 3067 in the "Number" box (or "needlestick safety" in the "Key word" box), and click on "GPO's PDF version of this bill."

Universal Precautions

OSHA follows the Centers for Disease Control and Prevention (CDC) guidelines for Universal Precautions, requiring the employer and employee to assume blood and other body fluids from any and all patients are infectious and therefore must be handled accordingly.

Engineering Controls and Work Practice Controls

Employers are required to provide hand-washing facilities readily accessible to employees. It is the employer's responsibility to ensure employees wash their hands immediately after gloves and other protective garments are removed.

Contaminated needles and other contaminated sharps shall not be bent, recapped, or removed unless the employer can demonstrate that no alternative is feasible or that a specific medical procedure requires such action. Recapping or needle removal must be accomplished by a mechanical device or a one-handed technique. Contaminated reusable sharps shall be placed in appropriate containers until properly processed. These containers must be puncture resistant, leak-proof, and labeled or color-coded in accordance with the regulations for easy identification.

Eating, drinking, smoking, applying cosmetics or lip balm, and handling contact lenses are prohibited in work areas where there is a reasonable likelihood of exposure to potentially infectious materials.

Food and drink must not be kept in refrigerators, freezers, shelves, cabinets, or on counter tops where blood or other potentially infectious or dangerous materials are present.

All procedures involving blood or other infectious materials shall be performed in a manner to minimize splashing, spraying, spattering, and creating droplets.

Specimens of blood or other potentially infectious materials must be placed in closed containers that prevent leakage during collection, handling, processing, storage, transport, or shipping. Containers must be labeled or color-coded in accordance with the regulations. If outside contamination of the primary container occurs, it must be placed within a second container that is leakproof, puncture resistant, and labeled or color-coded accordingly.

Personal Protective Equipment

Employers are required to provide appropriate personal protective equipment at no cost to employees whose job duties expose them to blood and other infectious materials. Appropriate personal protective equipment includes, but is not limited to, gloves, gowns, laboratory coats, face shields or masks, and eye protection. Personal protective equipment is considered appropriate if it prevents blood and other infectious materials from reaching the employee's work clothes, skin, eyes, mouth, or other mucous membranes under normal conditions of use.

Personal protective equipment in the appropriate sizes must be accessible at the work site or issued to employees. If a garment is penetrated by blood or other infectious materials, it must be removed immediately or as soon as possible. All personal protective equipment must be removed before leaving the work area.

Masks in combination with goggles or protective eye shields must be worn whenever splashes, spray, splatter, or droplets may be created and eye, nose, or mouth contamination can be reasonably anticipated, and face masks should be liquid resistant. Gloves and other protective body clothing shall be worn in occupational exposure situations. The type and characteristics will depend on the task and degree of exposure anticipated. Surgical caps or hoods and shoe covers must be worn in situations where gross contamination can be reasonably anticipated.

Employers must ensure the employee uses appropriate personal protective equipment unless the employer can demonstrate the employee temporarily declined to use the equipment, when under rare and extraordinary circumstances, it was the employee's professional judgment use of personal protective equipment would have prevented the delivery of healthcare services or would have posed an increased hazard to the safety of the worker or a co-worker. When an employee makes this judgment, the circumstances will be investigated and documented to determine whether changes can be made to prevent such situations in the future.

Gloves must be worn when it can be reasonably anticipated the employee may have contact with blood or other infectious materials to the hands, mucous membranes, and nonintact skin when performing vascular access procedures and when touching or handling contaminated surfaces.

Hepatitis B Vaccination

Employers are required to provide the hepatitis B vaccination free of charge to all employees who are at risk for occupational exposure. The vaccine must be provided within 10 days of an employee's initial assignment, except in cases where the employee has previously received the complete vaccination series, where antibody testing has revealed the employee is immune, or where the vaccine is contraindicated for medical reasons. Employees who refuse the vaccination must sign a Hepatitis B Vaccination Declination form. The employee, however, is allowed to change his or her mind and elect to receive the vaccine at any time at the employer's expense.

Post-Exposure Evaluation and Follow-Up

Following a report of an exposure incident, the employer must make immediately available to the exposed employee a confidential medical evaluation and follow-up, including at least the following:

- Documentation of the route(s) of exposure and the circumstances under which the exposure occurred.
- Identification and documentation of the individual who is the source of the blood or potentially infectious material, unless the employer can establish that identification is not feasible or is prohibited by state or local law. The source individual's blood shall be tested as soon as possible and after consent is obtained in order to determine HBV, HCV, or HIV infectivity. If consent is not obtained, the employer must document that legally required consent cannot be obtained. If the source individual's consent is not required by law, the source individual's blood, if available, shall be tested and the results documented. In cases where the source individual is already known to be infected, blood testing is not required. Results of the source individual's blood test shall be made available to the exposed employee, and the employee shall be informed of all applicable laws concerning the disclosure of the source individual's identity and infectious status.
- Collection and testing of the exposed employee's blood for HBV, HCV, and HIV status as soon as possible after the employee gives consent. If the employee consents to baseline blood collection but

does not give consent at that time for HIV testing, the sample shall be preserved for 90 days. Testing of the blood shall take place within the 90 days if the employee decides to do so.

- Post-exposure prophylaxis when medically indicated, as recommended by the Public Health Service.
- Counseling.
- Evaluation of reported illnesses. The employer must provide the employee with a copy of the evaluating health professional's written opinion within 15 days of completion. The written opinion shall be limited to the following:
  - Whether HBV vaccination is indicated for the employee and if the employee has received such vaccination.
  - The employee has been informed of the results of the evaluation.
  - The employee has been told about any medical conditions resulting from exposure to blood or other potentially infectious materials that require further evaluation or treatment.

All other findings or diagnoses must remain confidential and shall not be included in the written report.

Communication of Hazards to Employees

Warning labels must be on containers, refrigerators, and freezers containing blood or other potentially infectious materials and must be affixed to containers used to store, transport, or ship blood or other potentially infectious materials. The warnings must be fluorescent orange or orange-red; red bags or containers may be substituted for labels.

Employee training must be provided by the employer at no cost and during working hours at the time of initial assignment and at least annually thereafter. The training must include, at a minimum, the following:

- An explanation of the basis for selection of personal protective equipment.
- Information on the types, proper use, location, removal, handling, decontamination, and disposal of personal protective equipment.
- An explanation of the methods that will prevent or reduce exposure, including engineering controls, work practice controls, and personal protective equipment.

- Information on the HBV vaccine and vaccination free of charge.
- The procedure for follow-up after an exposure incident.
- Information on the post-exposure evaluation and follow-up the employer is required to provide.
- A copy of the Bloodborne Pathogen Regulations and an explanation of their contents. A general explanation of the epidemiology and symptoms of blood-borne diseases and an explanation of their modes of transmission.
- An explanation and a copy of the employer's exposure control plan.
- How to identify tasks and activities that may involve exposure.
- Appropriate actions to take and persons to contact in an emergency involving blood or other potentially infectious materials.
- Explanation of the signs and labels and color-coding requirements.
- An opportunity for interactive questions and answers with the person conducting the training session.

Required Record Keeping

The employer shall maintain for each employee at risk an accurate record of the following:

- Name and social security number
- Hepatitis B vaccination status
- Results of examinations, testing, and follow-up procedures performed
- Copy of health professional's written evaluations following an exposure incident
- Copies of information provided to health professional following an exposure incident

The employer shall ensure confidentiality of employee records. Information shall not be disclosed without the employee's written consent. The employer must maintain records for the duration of employment plus 30 years. The employer must maintain records of the training sessions for three years from the date of the training sessions, and these records shall include dates, names, and qualifications of persons who conducted training sessions and names and job titles of employees who attended.

ADDITIONAL RESOURCES

Exposure Prevention

Advances in Exposure Prevention is a publication for the prevention of occupational transmission of bloodborne pathogens. Published by the International Health Care Worker Safety Research and Resource Center at the University of Virginia. For subscriber information, call customer service at 804-924-5159; or visit the web site at http://www.med.virginia.edu/epinet.

EPINet (Exposure Prevention Information Network) And EPINet-OR are used for recording and sharing information on percutaneous injuries and blood and body fluid contacts to assist with OSHA's record-keeping requirements and to identify successful prevention measures. For information, call 804-982-0702.

Post-Exposure Follow-Up and Prophylaxis

For the most up-to-date information, contact National Clinicians' Post-Exposure Prophylaxis Hotline (PEPLine) at 1-888-HIV-4911 (1-888-448-4911). Twenty-four hours a day, seven days a week free state-of-the-art consultations for clinicians caring for healthcare workers who have sustained occupational exposures to blood and other potentially infectious body fluids.

PEPNet: Treatment protocols for clinicians treating exposed healthcare workers are available on the Internet at http://epi-center.ucsf.edu. Additional topics are available: When to Offer PEP, Choosing a PEP Regimen, Answers to Questions Frequently Asked by Exposed Healthcare Workers, Answers to Questions Frequently Asked by Clinicians Managing Occupational Exposures to HIV, Quick Reference to Anti-Retroviral Drug Adverse Effects and Drug-Drug interactions, Quick Reference to Anti-Retroviral Drug Use in Pregnancy, Post-Exposure Care for Hepatitis C Virus (HCV) Exposures.

The Centers for Disease Control and Prevention (CDC) has updated information on HIV post-exposure prophylaxis and exposure to HCV at http://www.cdc.gov.

The OSHA bloodborne pathogen standard documents and compliance directives are available at http://www.osha.org

GLOSSARY

AIDS—disease complex of opportunistic infections caused by the human immunodeficiency virus (HIV).

Anti-retroviral medications—drugs used for post-exposure prophylaxis against HIV and for the treatment of AIDS.

Bloodborne exposure—*see* Exposure, bloodborne

Continuous quality improvement (CQI)—continuously upgrading the safety of the working environment (generally improving services and controlling costs) by assembling a team, identifying problems, choosing and applying interventions, and measuring results.

Engineering controls—safety engineered devices intended for hazard abatement.

Exposure, bloodborne—contact with blood or body fluids contaminated with blood with the potential for transmission of disease from patient to healthcare worker.

Exposure, mucocutaneous—contact of health care workers' mucous membranes or nonintact skin with blood or body fluids contaminated with blood with the potential for transmission of disease from patient to healthcare worker.

Exposure, percutaneous—contact of health care workers' punctured or nonintact skin with blood or body fluids contaminated with blood with the potential for transmission of disease from patient to healthcare worker.

Exposure, surgical—contact between blood of the surgeon or other member of the surgical team and the surgical patient's internal tissues.

Hazard abatement—reduction of occupational risk of injury or exposure to blood and body fluids.

HBIG—hepatitis B immune globulin.

HBV—hepatitis B.

HCV—hepatitis C.

HDV—hepatitis D.

HGV—hepatitis G.

HICPAC—Hospital Infection Control Practices Advisory Committee.

HIV—human immunodeficiency virus.

Lamivudine (3TC)—drug used in combination with zidovudine (ZDV) for HIV post-exposure prophylaxis.

Mucocutaneous exposure—*see* Exposure, mucocutaneous

Nonresponders—persons not producing sufficient antibody for protection against hepatitis B following vaccination.

Neutral Zone (also Safe Zone)—a device or designated area of the sterile field in which sharps are placed, accessed, returned, and retrieved to avoid hand-to-hand transfer of sharps between personnel.

OSHA (Occupational Safety and Health Administration)—federal agency charged with ensuring a healthy and safe work environment.

Percutaneous exposure (PE)—see Exposure, percutaneous

Percutaneous injury (PCI)—a cut, needlestick, or other injury.

Personal protective equipment (PPE)—apparel or devices worn to prevent exposures to blood and other infectious materials.

PCR (polymerase chain reaction)—direct measurement of viral DNA used to test for HIV and hepatitis C where antibody testing may be inaccurate, especially shortly after occupational exposure.

Post-exposure management—follow-up and treatment of exposed persons following blood and body fluid exposure.

Post-exposure prophylaxis (PEP)—administration of anti-retroviral drugs in various combinations as considered appropriate according to updated guidelines following significant exposure to HIV.

Precautions, Advanced—Proposed by the author in 1999: Bloodborne exposure prevention, in invasive settings, based on effectively selecting and using the most appropriate and up-to-date techniques and technology, monitored, maintained and upgraded by continuous quality improvement (CQI). For example, double-gloving using the most effective (and cost-effective) glove combinations.

Precautions, Standard—issued by the CDC and HICPAC in 1996: Combines Universal Precautions and Body Substance Isolation, which is designed to reduce the risk of transmission of pathogens from moist body substances. Standard Precautions apply to blood, *all* body fluids, secretions, and excretions *except* sweat regardless of whether they contain visible blood, nonintact skin, and mucous membranes. Standard Precautions are designed to reduce the risk of transmission of microorganisms from both recognized and unrecognized sources of infection in hospitals. (*Am J Infect Control* 1996;24:24–52.)

Precautions, Universal—issued by the CDC in 1985: Applying Blood and Body Fluid Precautions (use of gloves, gowns, masks and eye coverings, needlestick prevention) universally to all persons regardless of their presumed infection status. Replaces Isolation Precautions. For example, wearing gloves during all procedures where exposure to blood or any other body fluid may occur. Universal Precautions also require hand washing after glove removal.

Protease inhibitors—class of drugs used in the treatment of patients with AIDS and as a third drug for HIV post-exposure prophylaxis in high-risk exposures.

Recontact—*see* Exposure, surgical

Safety Champion—project coordinator/facilitator

Safe Zone—(see Neutral Zone)

Sharps—devices with a sharp point, blade, or edge, which may cause injury.

Sharps injury—*see* Percutaneous injury

Surgical exposure—*see* Exposure, surgical

Universal Precautions—*see* Precautions, Universal

Viral load (Viral Count)—the number of viruses per milliliter of blood.

Work practice controls—protocols and policies to prevent exposures.

INDEX